THE MINDSET OF A
MENTAL PATIENT
(AND A FEW LIGHTER ASIDES)
A PERSONAL POETIC JOURNEY
THROUGH THE MENTAL HEALTH
MINEFIELD

D1796248

Christopher J. Fairweather

'One million people commit suicide every year'
The World Health Organization

Christopher J. Fairweather

Published by
Chipmunkapublishing
PO Box 6872
Brentwood
Essex CM13 1ZT
United Kingdom

http://www.chipmunkapublishing.com

Edited by Shareen Ali

www.christopherfairweather.com

Cover Image by Jemimah Kuhfeld

(www.jemimahkuhfeld.co.uk).

Thank you and dedications.

There are many people I would like to thank for helping me though the last nine years of my life. First of all to my family for always being there for me, through some very troubled times, most importantly my mum, dad, my Grandmother, my sister and her husband James. Also just as importantly I would like to thank all the medical people who have looked after me through the years, all the Doctors and Community Nurses who were indispensable to me, the mental health team at Loughborough University, and my psychiatrist in Loughborough for giving me encouragement and helping answer a lot of questions about myself. Also, I would like to thank my friends, Audrey, and Sandy & Tom, and Susie, Melody, Richard and Ruth for always being kind and wonderful company and all the friends I have made though performing my poems at the various venues I have always been made so welcome at. I would also like to thank everyone at the various places I have worked at who were so understanding about my problems and making my life easier than it otherwise would have been. From Bristol I would like to thank my landlady for giving me a place to live in Bristol when luck was not on my side, and also to Ben for listening to my confused ranting before I sought medical help, and Ed for helping me so much in my final year. I would also like to thank everyone at Loughborough University for helping me through my degree there and giving me a year, which would have been much more difficult had they not been so helpful and accommodating to me. Finally, I would like to thank God for putting up with my moaning and keeping me safe through all of my many worries.

I would like to dedicate this book to my Nan and Granddad.

Contents

Christopher J. Fairweather

Introduction

I was first hit with mental health problems when I went to university in 1998. I went to study for a BA (Hons) in Business Administration at the University of the West of England in Bristol. Some months prior to leaving for Bristol my problems started. I decided to read the Bible. I had always believed in God, but I was not what you could call a model Christian, and I had decided that I wanted to change my ways. I found the bible in parts very enlightening and liberating, but also in places rather frightening due to the punishments the Bible mentions in places, and it was that which would prove my undoing and the start of my troubles. For anyone who is wondering, I am still a Christian and in many ways have come out of my trauma a stronger and (I hope) a more reasonable person. However, the last 9 years have often been very black, and not just for religious reasons as some problems I have had with mental health have lead to other problems further along the way.

This book takes you on the journey of the last 9 years my life through poems, and through these poems, I hope to show what living with mental health problems is like. One in four of us shall experience mental health problems during their life, and yet the misunderstanding, discrimination, stigmatization and intolerance of people with mental health problems continue. Many people with mental health problems (myself included) find it very difficult to find employment. Many employers demand to know if people applying for jobs have mental health problems, and in a survey referred to by the BBC on the 10/10/06 revealed that 2/3 of employers are reluctant to employ people with mental health problems, and 33% of people with mental health problems claim they have been sacked or forced to resign when they have declared their condition to their employer.

With statistics like these, it is really a catch-22 situation for people such as myself. If we declare mental health problems on a job application form we are protected by employment law, but a prejudiced employer can often find another reason not to employ us, and if we do not declare anything and are subsequently found out, we risk dismissal from our job.

The spectrum of mental health problems is broad and it is wide, but the ignorance of many people about these problems means so often that all of us with mental problems (including myself) are just branded as psychos, loonies or nuts, and we are not given a fair chance. I have been reasonably lucky in being accepted by people I have met in my life when I have told them about my problems, but others are not so lucky, and this book also partly shows what it is like to live with the prejudice that goes on.

However, the journey is not all doom and gloom. Over the years, I have written some other poems about other subjects, and I have included these poems in order to lighten up the journey. I hope you enjoy them.

To begin, here is an overview of how my problems started:

Christopher J. Fairweather

CHAPTER ONE

SCHOOL DAYS

The Stolen Bible

When I was in lessons at school one day,
A teacher told me what he had to say.

He said:
"Take this bible that's been left here,
And return it to the store room near."
But instead of that, I took it home,
And read every single page alone,
To try and please God and know him well,
But instead, I was teetering on the rim of hell.

For then my problems began to begin,
As I tried to live my life without sin,
And a verse about the Holy Ghost
Did scramble my brain and mind the most.

It said:
Do not speak evil of this Great Being,
For everything you do, the Good Lord is seeing,

And if you speak evil, God will ring a great bell,
To signify that you are bound for hell.

So I tried my very best to be good to the Spirit,
But very soon, my brain just wasn't with it.
It was its own brain and it was its own mind,
And to my conscience it was so unkind,
For in trying to be good I made mistakes that were bad,
And very soon, my life was all very sad.
With hindsight, I could have used a scold's bridle,
And very soon, I was suicidal.

I said:
"Doctor, please help me, my brain is a mess,
Can you give me some tablets?"
My Doctor said "Yes", and
"I will set the wheels in motion too,
To get permanent help for your mind and for you."

So through the years I did push on,
Though I often wished my life was totally gone,
But the thought of that wish was always allied
To the fact, I'd go to hell if I committed suicide.

I said:
"Father, please help me, take my problems away,
And banish my paranoia in some way."
But the fear stayed with me and made moves which were bold,
And to this day leaves my conscience out in the cold.

THE MINDSET OF A MENTAL PATIENT

So ten years later, and I'm still here,
Though I often wish that the end were near,
For all my paranoid problems, up to me they sidle,
And all because I stole that Bible.

Though I did not realize it at the time, that day
when I was given this Bible would change my life
forever. It is true to say that my problems did
escalate when I read the Bible, but I do not blame
religion for my problems. In some ways it was an
extension of a condition I have had since I was a
baby, but did not find out about until 2006. This
condition is known as Asperger's Syndrome.

Asperger's Syndrome has been described as
'having a dash of autism.' Many sufferers can
have specialist skills in many fields such as being
brilliant artists, writers and many other things as
well, but we often come across as rather
eccentric, strange or slightly weird or as loners.
The condition was not officially recognized until
1993, and before this time many sufferers were
simply thought of as eccentric, but if you want to
be accepted at school, eccentric is not the thing to
be. At school in order to fit in you often have to be
'cool.' This was something I was never interested
in being, and I would say as much to my peers.
This with hindsight was perhaps not the best thing
to do, and I got a lot of stick and was bullied a lot
because of it. This next poem sums up how I felt
and how I was treated because of my views:

Uncool and Proud of It

I'm uncool and proud of it,
I believe that's the way.
I'm uncool and proud of it,
And that's how I'll stay,
For in coolness there's sneering
And pressure to conform
To be things you don't want to be,
And that is the norm.

To be cool at school,
You have to act like your peers,
Or endure their taunting,
Like I did for years.
But they were the cool ones,
And they caused all the trouble,
And as I wouldn't conform
They reduced me to rubble.

But they didn't succeed
In making me live life their way.
"I'm uncool" I shouted,
"And that's how I'll stay.
I'll do the things I want to,
Not just what's cool,
I'll live life my own way,
And not to your rule.
So please say I'm an anorak,
I really don't care,
If I want to stare at trains,
I'll do it, SO THERE.
I'm not hurting your lives

THE MINDSET OF A MENTAL PATIENT

By doing what I do,
So why do you bully me?
What's in it for you?

And you're not going to break me,
No matter how hard you try.
I do the things I want
While you live a lie.
You might make me feel sad,
But I won't give in,
And no matter how you try,
You will not win."

So I'm uncool and proud of it,
And will be forever,
While those who want cool
Are at the end of their tether,
Trying to keep up
With whatever's in fashion,
Even though deep down
They hate it with a passion.

I say,
"Join the uncool army,
We do what we please.
We don't taunt all others
To bring them to their knees.
We just get on with what we want,
And so could you."
And if the we all did that,
We'd all be happier too.

Whilst some of my classmates were happy to let

me be me, others were not. I was regularly bullied, normally verbally and this made me even more of a loner, which in turn led me to be bullied.

Even at this stage in my life, I could see that other people saw me a rather weird. My stammer did not help me fit in either, although oddly (and happily) are almost never got bullied about that.

One form of negativity I got used to over the years was if I met a new pupil for the first time. I would introduce myself in what I considered to be a normal way, but within no more than a few minutes of talking to me, often the new pupil would fix with me with a look, a look I got very used to, which said 'You are WEIRD!!)

At the time I never knew why they did this, and I wouldn't until many years later.

What I did know was that I certainly didn't fit in, but in a funny way I liked the fact that I didn't fit in. I didn't like all the stick I got for being weird and for not being cool, and life at school was often not enjoyable. But I decided that if it was the price I had to pay for not fitting in, I would rather pay it than conform to the teenage tribal instinct and buy clothes I didn't want to wear, books I didn't want to read and music I didn't want to listen to just to be accepted.

As you can see, my school days were not always the happiest of my life, but as time has passed I have come to realize how important they were in shaping me and making me what I am now. However, I did not realize that at the time.

Another thing I did not realize was that my problems were only beginning, because when I went away to University, things would get much worse.

Christopher J. Fairweather

CHAPTER TWO

A SPANNER IN THE WORKS

As I discussed in the introduction, and in the poem, The Stolen Bible, my problems began after I read a passage of the Bible, which stated that anyone who speaks evil of the Holy Spirit has committed eternal sin and will never be forgiven. This frightened me. Ever since I was young, I had always been a total worry-guts and as my teenage life continued, I became more and more paranoid with the passing of time.

Whilst few poems exist of my time at university, I recount here the story of my time there in order that the rest of the book makes sense.

The comedian Ben Elton in the 1980s had done a routine called Captain Paranoia. His idea was that we all have an invisible demon that lives our shoulder called Captain Paranoia, and that this malignant being messes around with your brain making you paranoid and worried all the time. His examples include being in church at a friend's wedding when the vicar comes to the part where he says,

"Does any one know of any reason why these two cannot wed?"

It is here that the paranoia takes over and makes you fear that you are about to go mad and shout out that you know of a reason when of course you don't know of one.

When I heard this routine, I immediately identified with it. There was no doubt about it, paranoia was with me, and when I read this passage about the Holy Spirit in the Bible, though I did not realize it at the time the die had been cast for what the next nine years of my life would be like.

As time passed in the summer of 1998, I realized that in order to stop myself saying or thinking inappropriate things about the Holy Spirit, I had to distract my mind by saying and thinking nice things about it. To start with I did not find this too much of a problem. I had left school by now and the only responsibility I had was my part-time job at Tesco, and life was reasonably happy, until I went away to University at the University of the West of England in Bristol.

Shortly after arriving in Bristol, things started to go downhill fast. I was still having to distract my mind by saying and thinking nice things about the Holy Spirit, and whilst up until now it had been quite easy, the stresses of living away from home for

THE MINDSET OF A MENTAL PATIENT

the first time living in a strange town with housemates I didn't know, and doing something that nothing in life had prepared me for tipped me over the edge. I started to make mistakes when I was trying to say and think nice things of the Holy Spirit, and sometimes inadvertently said or thought nasty things about it. The first time it happened I was lying on my bed in my room, words buzzing around my head, and suddenly, I said something wrong, and this is really, where the problems started.

Over the following weeks and months, I became very depressed and suicidal. My brain kept making the mistakes. I was scared that I had committed this terrible eternal sin. I started hearing voices. Things went from bad to worse. I did not know who to turn to or what to do.

Throughout this period, one of my housemates was concerned about me. When I would come home late at night from my part-time job, always distressed and confused, he would be happy to talk and he would try to reassure me. With hindsight I'm not sure if he really liked me, and in the state I was in I wouldn't blame him if he didn't, but he was prepared to listen to my problems and try to offer help. If you are reading this, Ben, I would like to thank you for what you did for me. You were a great help.

One day in 1999, things came to a head. In a weak moment, I drove my car to the deserted top storey of a car park in Bristol. I parked the car, got out, walked to the edge of the car park and looked over the edge. I was wondering about jumping. I thought that the rest of my life was going to be like this, and that if I was going to Hell anyway, what was the point of prolonging my agony on earth? But as I stood there, I heard a voice, a voice that I had not heard before and on very few occasions since. It was different to all of the other voices that I had been hearing. It was just saying one word over and over again. It just said in a calm whisper:

"No."

I stood there in a daze, not sure of what I was thinking and with my heart thumping. The voice continued, still just saying "no". I started to think; "Is this God telling me not to jump?" After some thought I could not think of any other explanation for it. I decided not to jump and gradually I began to calm down and my heartbeat returned to normal.

This was another turning point in my life. As I began to walk away from the edge of the car park and began to descend from the top storey of the car park to the ground floor so that I could walk in to the town I decided that I had to seek professional help for how I was feeling, and this I did.

However, that is not the full story. Before I had left

THE MINDSET OF A MENTAL PATIENT

home for Bristol, the university had advised me (as they did for all 1st year students) to register with a doctor in Bristol, however I had never done this, thinking that as I had never had much call for medical help up until now, I would be OK. With hindsight, I am glad I hadn't signed on with a doctor in Bristol, because my failure to do this meant that I would have to visit my family's doctor in Romsey, which was the town close to where we lived. Whilst I had not had a huge amount of contact with this doctor, he did at least know me better than a doctor in Bristol would have done, and as I will tell you later, there was another important reason that visiting this doctor would have benefits for me.

The day of my visit to the doctor came round. I left Bristol early in the morning to make the long journey to Romsey. I arrived at the surgery and waited in the waiting room, trying to work out the best way to articulate the problems I was having so he would understand. After a few minutes, I was called in.

"What can I do for you?" he asked.

"I am hearing voices and I feel very depressed," I told him.

I then proceeded to tell him everything I have told you above. I told him about the passage in the Bible and how in a roundabout way it had led me to end up in the mess I was now in. I also told him about a flashback that I had had shortly after my flirtation with suicide. I had come home late one night, depressed as usual and I had explained my troubles to my very understanding housemate, Ben. Whilst I was talking about how I was feeling suicidal, I imagined myself standing on top of the car park, just as it had happened, but then my mind had taken over. Without me thinking about it, I saw this mental picture of myself suddenly climb over the wall on the top floor of the car park, and for a short time, I actually felt the sensation of the wind rushing past my face as I hurtled down towards the ground. Then the vision disappeared. I had found this very frightening.

My doctor was most understanding about my problems, and immediately set the wheels in motion for me to see a psychiatrist. More by luck than judgment, I had timed my visit to my doctor very well. In a month or so, I would be coming towards the end of my 1st year exams, and I would be able to return home for the summer break and receive permanent treatment.

At the end of the appointment, about 45 minutes later, I suddenly realized that my clothes were saturated with sweat. I felt my brow. The sweat was cold. Up until now, I thought that it was a myth that people got cold sweats, but I was dripping from head to foot. I thanked my doctor and left the surgery.

My doctor had given me a prescription for some

medication, and this is where the other benefit I told you about came in. I had been prescribed Olanzapine for my condition, which then a very new (and very expensive) drug, which did not have many of the harmful side effects that older drugs that are used for treating mental health problems have. Back then, I did not realize know the full details of the 'postcode lottery' as it is called, but if I had registered with a doctor in Bristol and gone to him with my problems, there is a chance that I would have been prescribed one of these older drugs.

Over the following weeks, I managed to get through my exams in Bristol. Over this period, I also saw a psychiatrist and was put in the care of a Community Nurse (the first was called Stuart and later I had one called Martin. I found their help invaluable to me, and the many meetings that I had had with them had been a lifeline to me, and if either of you are reading this I would like to publicly thank you both for all the assistance you gave me during what was a very troubled time of my life.

Both of these lifelines were very helpful to me, and whilst they obviously did not cure my problems, it was invaluable to have the support and have people who would listen to my paranoid worries and problems without thinking that I was barking mad, and whilst my fight against my problems was by no means easy, it certainly made the hill I was climbing less steep.

However, I was still hearing the voices, I was still making mistakes, and I was often feeling suicidal. Throughout this time, I was praying to God daily, and asking Him to end my life if I could not be forgiven for what I had done before I caused Him any more problems. In my confused state of thinking that I was going to go to Hell, I sometimes wondered if some of the voices that I was hearing were coming from the Devil. One night, after another bad evening at work, where I had made several mistakes regarding the Holy Spirit, I was walking through the warehouse where a voice, different from the one I had heard on top of the car park said just one word:

"Good-bye."

I was distressed by this, and at first thought it was Jesus losing patience with me and leaving me for good, having decided to send me to Hell when I died. But then I thought again. This voice was different from the one I heard on the car park, and I had never heard this voice before. I had heard it said that the Devil prayed on the weak, and at this time, I certainly was weak. I then thought that this might be a trick on the part of the Devil, trying to make me think that God was leaving me. One of the things which had ultimately deterred be from committing suicide was my *personal* belief that I would go to Hell if I did, and maybe this was an attempt on the part of the Devil to trick me into committing suicide. A few weeks later, I think I found the answer.

THE MINDSET OF A MENTAL PATIENT

These few weeks went by, and in the summer of 1999 (as I did every year), I would go on holiday and visit my mother's family who all lived in the village of Caister-on-Sea in Norfolk. It was a wonderful set-up. My Nan and Granddad lived in one house, and the sister of my Mother lived next door with her husband and two children (my cousins).

Whilst I was still feeling depressed at this time, I loved Norfolk. My Nan was a wonderful person I enjoyed her company enormously. The sad thing was that though I did not realize this at the time, this would be the last time I would see her, as she would sadly die before I got to visit her again. But as you will see later, the last thing she did for me was the most important thing that she ever did, and Nan, if you are able to look down to see me writing this, I thank you for it, and all of the wonderful times I had with you and Grandad together.

It was on this visit to Norfolk that I found the answer to my question. One afternoon I was sitting in my Cousin's bedroom, listening to a local Norfolk radio station. All was normal. After a while, he left the room for a few minutes, and whilst he was out of the room something happened which I am sure I didn't imagine, and at that, time chilled me to the core. Suddenly a voice yelled out from the radio:

"THEY'RE'S NO-ONE COMING TO SAVE YOU,

YOU'RE FINISHED!"

There was now no doubt in my mind; this was the Devil who was out to get me, trying to make me believe I was finished, that I was going to Hell and that nothing would stop this from happening.

My mind stewed with this problem for a few hours, and then I returned to my Nan's house for the evening, and wrote the first of many poems I would write about my mental health problems, and here it is:

A Poem from the Depths of Depression (circa 1999)

As I search for the answers,
I know not if they come.
They might do or they mightn't do,
My brain is going numb.

A voice screams from the radio,
A message or just a jingle?
The former I might as well be dead,
The latter I'm just still single.

In life I've had it easy.
I've never starved inside,
But I find it really hard
To find the will to stay alive.

Some people just dance through,
As if all, their days are sun,

THE MINDSET OF A MENTAL PATIENT

By I just crawl from one to another
In my mental slum.

Could jumping be the answer?
If I'm destined to go down,
Or is 60 years of earth hell worth it
Before I finally drown?

In life I've had it easy,
I've never starved inside,
But I find it really hard
To find the will to stay alive.

I've found the help that's out there,
Though life's not an easy ride,
But they do their best to help me
Find the will to stay alive.

I'll try to trust in God at all times,
And my medicine for a high,
And the moments of relief, I find
From a midnight turquoise sky.

This poem sums up how I felt at the time. My
tablets were helping me to keep going, and now
that I felt that the Devil was out to try and get me, I
felt I had little to lose by trying trust in God.

It was at times like this in the depressed state I
was in then, and have been in at times since as
well, that little innocuous things than help lift the
mood. Leaving work late one night, I saw the sky
a colour I had never seen it before. And for some

reason that I cannot explain, this made me feel a little better about the future, although I held out little hope of it being plain sailing, and a few weeks later, I was to be proved right.

A few days before the end of my holiday, I told my Nan about my problems, and little silly things that were getting the better of me. I had become scared of the number 666 after reading it in the Book of Revelations. Since my problems had started, for some reason I had got it into my head that if I saw this number anywhere, on a car number plate, in a telephone number or in a VideoPlus code, or anywhere else it was a calling card from the Devil, just to serve as a reminder that he hadn't forgotten about me.

My Nan was most understanding. All her life she had been a Christian and was a worker and fund-raiser for the local Church. She arranged for me to meet the Vicar of the Parish, which I did. He did his best to reassure me, explaining that sinning against the Holy Spirit mentioned in the Bible was in fact, impossible. This gave me hope. Whilst it did not take my fears away, it certainly made me feel better. We talked at length and I left, still feeing worried, but much happier about things than I had been for a while.

Shortly after this, my holiday ended, and I left Norfolk having said good-bye to my relatives, and, as it would turn out, for the last time to my Nan. I was feeling a little better. I was traveling straight

THE MINDSET OF A MENTAL PATIENT

to Bristol from Norfolk to set up home in my new house for my second year at University, but for reasons that will become apparent, my new house would very soon turn into a nightmare that still affects me to this day.

Prior to leaving Bristol for the summer break after my 1st year exams, I had had to organize my accommodation for my 2nd year. For the first year at the university, you were given accommodation owned by the university, but for the second and final years, you had to find your own in the private sector. Fortunately, (as it seemed), I had found somewhere.

During my first year, I had regularly attended small communion services on the campus centre for religious affairs, which was called the Octagon. Over the months, I had got to know a girl there and we got on quite well. I had mentioned my condition to her, and as we came to the end of the academic year, I mentioned that I was looking for accommodation. At this point, I had found a potential house, and was looking for other people to move in with. She mentioned to me that she already had a house, but was looking for others to move in with her because her three current housemates were soon graduating. I went round to look at the house, and it was nice. I subsequently contacted the landlord, and we agreed terms.

The start of my 2nd year came around, and I

moved into the new house. We were shortly joined by two other students, also Christian. All appeared to go well. I thought we were getting on, and they were all nice to me. I would sometimes talk briefly about my condition, and it did not seem to be a problem for them. What I did not realize was that it was all a façade. Really, they didn't like me, and soon I was to find out why.

One Thursday night I was the only one at home, and suddenly, totally unannounced, the landlord turned up, sat me down in the living room and told me in no uncertain terms that my housemates did not like me. Due to my mental health problems, they all thought I was strange, and that as of Friday he wanted me to find somewhere else to live. This came as a bolt from the blue to me. I had no idea that they felt this way. I pleaded to the landlord for time to talk it through with them; he reluctantly agreed and then left. When my housemates returned I tried to talk to them, but it was ultimately no use. They were decided. Over the next few days they showed me a letter they had sent to the landlord, saying that in their opinion, I had serious mental health problems and that they did not want to live with me. On the Sunday night, one of my housemates came into my room and talked to me. I was so scared and shattered. I was physically shaking. Whilst being ladylike about the problems, the deal I was offered was that either I leave the house of my own accord, or the three of them would. This I could not take. In the state I was in, I could not handle the guilt of forcing my housemates to find another house, so I said I would look for alternative accommodation. I really had no option. Stupidly, I had no contract with my landlord, so I had no rights.

Over the following week, I searched for new accommodation, and then I found what would indeed turn out to be the perfect place, living as lone lodger. The room was nice and the rent was very reasonable. After a short time, I made my decision to move there, and I'm very glad I did. My new landlady was a lovely lady, and was much more open-minded about my problems, and I would like to thank her publicly for taking me in when I was very much down on my luck. I enjoyed my time living with her, and if she is reading this now, thank you very much indeed.

Shortly after I decided to move in to her house, I made several journeys between what had become a hellhole and my new accommodation, in order to move my belongings. As I was sitting in my car, preparing to leave my old place for the final time, the girl I had originally met at the Octagon came to say goodbye.

"I'm sorry it hasn't worked out," she said.

"So am I," I said.

I said goodbye and drove away.

I drove away in two minds about something I had thought about saying as a parting shot, but did not. Part of me was wishing I had left after saying:

"And may God forgive you for not forgiving me!"

It was something, which I wish I had said, but I'm glad I didn't, if that is not a contradiction in terms. I might have enjoyed it at the time, but would have definately regretted it afterwards.

In my weakened mental health state at the time, however, there was a sense of injustice that I just could not get my head around. The four people I had spent my 1st year with in the university-owned house had been very nice people. With hindsight I am not certain if they actually liked me, but they had been prepared to live with me and my condition, and they had all been supportive and sympathetic towards it, before and after I had sought professional help. But there was one thing that seemed strange. When I say what I am about to say, I wish to emphasize that just because I am a Christian I claim no superiority (morally or in any other way) over anyone else of any other faith or of no faith, but in the state I was in at the time, there was something that I could not understand. My housemates in my 1st year as far as I could tell had not been particularly religious, and yet they had been sympathetic towards me. The three housemates I had met in my 2nd year had all been Christian, and they treated me like a leper after they learnt about my condition. If anything, I thought,(in a stereotypical sense at least) it should have been the other way round. But I had learnt a valuable lesson about one of the oldest clichés in the world, that of 'Don't judge a book by its cover,' and that people of no faith can be nicer than those who claim to be of a faith.

In the long run however, the episode made more open-minded and understanding of how people are all different, and although it was traumatic at the time, perhaps it has helped strengthened. The house I moved to was a much happier place to live in, and if I had continued living in the house I left, I daresay everything would have only got worse.

If any of my housemates from that brief period that was so difficult for all four of us are reading this, I am sorry for the problems I caused you, but at the same time from my end all is forgiven, I bear you no malice and I hope things have worked out well for you in the time that has passed since. Maybe if things like that hadn't happened, in the long run my life might not have worked out as happily.

....

The rest of my second year was uneventful by comparison, but my bad experience had left a scar on me and it led me to worry, for now I was now uncontrollably paranoid that if people I knew (students, lecturers, other staff, friends or workmates) were anything less than ecstatically happy with me, I thought I must have done something to offend them, in the same way I had troubled my housemates by being mentally ill. Deep down I knew the chances of my offending people were small, but paranoia is a powerful emotion, and it was not about to let me go free.

Coming towards the end of my 2nd year, it was the plan that I would do a one-year placement with a business somewhere in the UK as part of my course, but I was unable to find one. This was perhaps an example of many employers being reluctant to take on people with mental health problems, although I do realize that I was not the strongest student on the course.

I decided to take a year out from the course instead, and work for Tesco in Southampton doing various jobs. This year, although unhappy for all of the reasons discussed above also passed reasonably uneventfully, but when I returned to university for my final year, I would have an experience that whilst not (at the time) life changing, was wonderful, essential, and made me look at my faith in a new way.

CHAPTER THREE

A NEW GUIDING HAND

By the end of my year out, I was feeling considerably better than I had at the start, though I was still far from perfect. However, this was not to last. A few weeks before I returned to university for the start of my final year I had to go back to the campus to deliver some papers to them, and as soon as I set foot on the campus again, the feelings of depression, drudgery and fear returned when I knew that I was returning to face another year in an establishment I had come to associate with all the negativity it had brought me. But I knew I had to go back.

On the upside, I had been able to get in contact with the landlady I had rented my room from in my second year, and she was happy to have me back. This was a great weight of my mind as having had bad experiences of communal living in the past I had been dreading finding somewhere to live again, and I was overjoyed and relieved to know that I would be able to live on my own again with people I knew and liked.

I returned to the campus for the new academic year and it was no different from when I left at the end of my second year. The depression, drudgery and fear were with me constantly, and as time passed, I began to struggle with understanding the work. There was one compulsory module on the course that I simply could not get my head around. In the mindset I was in, if the lecturers had been speaking Japanese I might have had a better chance of understanding it. I would make notes in lectures without understanding a word of what I was writing down. At times like this, my mind wandered easily and I found it almost impossible to concentrate. I think this might have been one of the side effects of my medication, but I knew that there was no way I could stop taking that.

I struggled on, feeling that I was sinking deeper and deeper all the time. Sometimes I thought of packing it all in and becoming a monk, and on more than one occasion, I had looked on the Internet to try to find out more about trying to become one. But I did not know that things were about to change. It would not make everything in my life plain sailing, but I definitely know that what happened was essential to my successful completion of the course.

THE MINDSET OF A MENTAL PATIENT

One module I did like on my course and one, which I was quite good at, was called International Employment Relations. My lecturer and tutor, Dr. Martin Upchurch was a wonderful teacher, and in the tutorials, without wishing to sound a show-off, I sometimes ended up contributing to answers to his questions so often he would sometimes ask for other people to answer who were more shy about contributing instead.

It was at the end of one of these tutorials that everything changed. I was packing my books when another student, who I had never seen on the course before came over and started talking to me. He offered to help me with my university work, and we exchanged phone numbers. I was a little surprised he had come to me like this, and in the first week afterwards I made no contact with him, but the following week after the tutorial he came to me again. I do not remember exactly what he said, but the result was that we became good friends and started helping each other with the modules on our course that we had in common. Wonderfully, we balanced out well in the different areas of the course, I was better at some things than he was, and he was better at some things than I was. His name was Ed.

Over time, as we got to know each other better, I hesitantly told him about my problems, not knowing what to expect his response to be. He could not have been more understanding, and if anything, it brought us closer together. As time passed, we began the lengthy revision process for our final exams. The fact that we were both good at different subjects helped enormously with the revision. We would write revision notes for each other on the subjects that one of us was better at than the other one, and it was at this point that I started to understand better the material on some of the modules that I was struggling with. It was all thanks to Ed. We would meet almost daily in a quiet corner of the library, and go through what we had prepared for one another, and it was very enjoyable.

The exam sessions came around, and we both did our best. After my final exam, I said what turned out to be a final goodbye to Ed. We never meant to lose touch with one another, but after the results of the exams came out, unfortunately, we did, and the following year I think I might have found out the reason why, although it is not a reason many of you will be expecting.

The same day of my final exam, I packed up all of my belongings from Bristol and made the journey home. I said goodbye to my landlady, and I would like to thank her again here for being so nice and understanding to me during my time with her, and for having me back after my year out. I would have certainly found my years much harder if I had had to find accommodation elsewhere.

I returned home to begin the nervous wait for the exam results, and to try and find a job. As the day of the results drew ever closer I began to worry more and more. Had I understood the exam questions? Had I made any stupid mistakes? Had I left out any important points?

The day the results came, I was working at Tesco in Southampton. On my coffee break, I went to my locker and checked my mobile phone. There was one message on there. It was from Ed, who as he was still on the campus had agreed to text me my result. White with fear I opened the text. It said three words:

"2:2 old boy."

I had done it. I had suffered a breakdown, nearly committed suicide, been treated like a leper because of my mental health problems, and thought of packing it all in, BUT I HAD DONE IT! I telephoned my parents to tell them, and Ed to thank him. When I did, Ed revealed to me that he had to do a retake in one module. I felt very sorry for him. He had helped me so much and still the trial was not over for him. I wished him all the best for it, little knowing that I would never see him again. If you are reading this Ed, or if anyone is who knows him, please get in touch. I would love to meet you again to say thank you properly, although for reasons that will become apparent later, I believe there is a reason why I will never meet him again, not in this life anyway.

Over the following months, I worked at Tesco,

trying unsuccessfully trying to find full-time employment. Although I now had a 2:2 BA (Hons) in Business Administration, I was now not sure if that was the career path I wanted to pursue. I had learnt that the business world is very cutthroat, and whilst I am by no means perfect, having to knife other people in the back to get where I wanted to go was not something that I relished doing. I would eventually find employment as an Administration Assistant , but before I started that, I was going to attend my graduation ceremony at Bristol Cathedral.

The graduation day came around. I arrived at the Cathedral with my family, and got in the queue for my robes and to have my picture taken. I was hoping to see Ed there, but something, which happened whilst I was queuing for my photograph made the feeling of joy I had at getting my degree a little bit sour.

Whilst I was in the queue, I noticed a display of university T-Shirts that were on sale, including one, which was called the "Class of 2002". I looked for my name on it, and it was there, but then I looked for Ed's name. It was not there. This made me rather sad. Ed's help had been instrumental in getting me though my final year and the exams at the end of it, and it was very sad to see that he had not made it through, but a few months later, I possibly found out the reason why.

One Sunday evening in 2003, I was watching

THE MINDSET OF A MENTAL PATIENT

Songs of Praise, and they were talking about the subject of Guardian Angels. They interviewed a woman who prior to discovering her faith had been through a bad time. I cannot remember exactly what had happened to her, but she was at a very low ebb. The woman told a story of how she was walking home one day and had got to her street that was full of terraced houses. The street was deserted. She arrived at her gate and started walking up the path to her house when she heard a voice from behind her. She turned around. Standing at the gate was a man she had never seen before, and asked her to come to him, which she did. This man reassured her, saying that he knew she had been through some bad times, but that things would improve for her. If I remember rightly, the woman was surprised (as you would be) but she listened to him and thanked him. After he had finished, he turned and walked away up the street. The lady turned and started to walk up the path to her door, but after a few steps she turned and looked back to try and see him. He had disappeared and the street was once again deserted.

The woman being interviewed thought this had been her Guardian Angel coming to reassure her. This sent my mind into a whirl. I had not heard from Ed for months. His name had not been on the graduation t-shirt that I had seen, and sometime previously I had left a message on his phone and he had not replied. Could Ed have been my Guardian Angel? As I have told you, I had never remembered seeing him on my course before, totally unexpectedly, he had come across at the end of a tutorial to talk to me, and he had seemed to be very keen to get to know me. I have always believed in God and angels and an afterlife. In my troubles in my final year I had prayed to God for help regularly, and I started to think; had God sent my Guardian Angel to look after me to ensure that I was able to get through my final year?

Some of you reading this may think that I am bonkers, and you are perfectly entitled to your opinion. I may be wrong in my ideas. I certainly cannot prove them, but to me it makes a lot of sense. As I have said, if Ed or anyone who knows him is reading this, if you want to, please get in touch, as I would love to meet you again. However, my theories maybe true and it may have been my Guardian Angel in which case God I thank you forever.

CHAPTER FOUR

OUT INTO THE BIG WORLD

Of course, getting my degree was one thing, but finding a job was to prove to be quite another. After I left Bristol, I was able to get a job working on the checkouts at Tesco in Southampton. It was mind-numbingly dull, and sometimes scary. Part of my condition is that I am predisposed to paranoia, and I lived in fear of various problems. One was the fear of getting into trouble if I accidentally accepted a false signature on a receipt (this was before the days of chip and pin) and risking getting into trouble over it, likewise with accidentally selling alcohol to underage customers. This was a big problem because Trading Standards would often send underage children through to find out if a store was selling alcohol to them, and if caught, the checkout assistant in question would get a criminal record and a large fine, neither of which I relished. The two main problems with this were that I was (and still am) a hopeless judge of age and on one occasion I asked someone who was 27 for ID, which was most embarrassing, and the Tesco I worked in was in a somewhat rough area and I had heard stories of teenagers trying to buy alcohol turning very nasty if they were asked for ID that proved their age.

Whilst I did not enjoy working there, the 7 months I was, passed reasonably uneventfully, until I was able to get a job as an Administration Assistant. For 5 months, I worked there, and as at Tesco things passed reasonably uneventfully. However, quite early on in my time there I was sent to work in another office for a week because they were short staffed, and I enjoyed it there. I returned to my original base shortly afterwards, but I did not know at the time how much my new office would affect me in the future.

As I have said, I worked at the first office for 5 months, and then one day my manager came to me and told me I was going to be sent back to the new office I I had helped out in some months previously for 8 weeks, again as they were short-staffed. I was pleased. I had been getting into a bit of a mental rut, and I was glad of the change.

To cut a long story short, I ended up at this new office permanently, and for a while all was well, until a fateful day went a new temp arrived, and though I didn't know it at the time, her presence would change my life.

As I have said, for a while, all was well, but then I

started to believe that this temp was not being very talkative towards me, and all my memories of my experiences in Bristol came flooding back to me. Had I done something to offend her? Was she upset with me? Was I in trouble? As I was able to find out at the time, I hadn't, but very soon, in a tragic accident I would.

It was Friday the 9th of January 2004, and I had had a good day. I was getting ready to go home, and only the temp and I were in the office. We were having a conversation, and I wasn't really concentrating. Without realising it my head dropped slightly and for a few seconds I was looking directly at her chest. She was understandably offended and without saying anything else to me, she stormed out of the office. It was here that my problems really began. The paranoia set in. Would she complain about me? Would I get into trouble? Would I lose my job? How would I face my family? How would I find another job without a reference from my present employer? These questions and fears were on constant playback in my head. I couldn't stop worrying about it. I was much too scared to talk to her about for fear of making things worse. But there was also another problem, and a very embarrassing one. I was living in fear of losing my job, and all of sudden I could not look at any other woman in the department without being scared that they would be thinking I was looking at them inappropriately, and hence they might complain about me. Every day I went into work expecting to be called into my manager's office to be brought to account. Every time one of my managers said "Good Morning Tony" to me sounding anything less than ecstatically happy with me, it sounded like a declaration of war, and paranoia kicked into action, trying to convince me that I was done for. I was scared that word would get around the department about what had happened, and that every woman there would think that, I was some undesirable letch. I couldn't look at another woman without being fearful of my eyes uncontrollably darting in the wrong direction and then suffering the most dreadful consequences. I became a nervous wreck. Every time I went home for the weekend, I was unable to enjoy it. I would just spend 48 being scared out of mind that I would be for the chop when returned to work on Monday.

Fate seemed to be against me all the time. It seemed that I would get to just before going home on Friday, and some event would happen that made me scared for the whole weekend. Someone would speak to me in a less than ecstatic tone of voice and my paranoia would spend the whole weekend convincing me that I was done for. Almost always, my worries came to nothing, but I could not stop my brain from worrying about all of the possible outcomes they could lead to if they came to fruition. I became suicidal again. My life seemed to have no point or meaning. It seemed to be an endless cycle of coming into work, being scared that I was offending people all day, then going home to worry about what the consequences might be, of the of the offence I thought I might have caused by my actions. I spent my life worrying about the what-ifs, and having people I spoke to about my problems telling me not to worry. If only it was as easy as that.

Many people with mental health problems have problems with worrying. It can take over their lives, like it had with me.

The 9th of January 2004 will stay with me as another of those days that changed my life forever. Although this problem has lessened over the years, it continued (in different forms) for a long time.

However, in a weird way, help was at hand. A few months after the dreadful incident, which had caused all of my problems, I saw a Channel 4 documentary about the wonderful late comedian Les Dawson. It was about his unpublished diaries.

Prior to his stardom, Les had had a tough upbringing in the north of England followed by series of soul-destroying dead-end jobs and disappointments just when it looked like things were going to improve for him. During this period, he had kept a diary, and written poems about what he was going through. I do not know quite why, but this fired me to write poems about how I was coping (and sometimes not coping) with my mental health problems, and how I was feeling in the horrible situation that I found myself in.

I was definitely going through the blackest period of my life at this time. Life in Bristol had been bad quite a lot of the time, but never as bad as this. But I found that writing the poems helped. They did not take my problems away, but I always felt a little better having committed something to paper. Many of my early poems had a similar theme; here are two examples:

Worrying About the What-Ifs.

I spend my life worrying about what-ifs,
For some time, it's been this way.
People tell me, "Just stop it".
It's easy for them to say.

Don't they think that if I could stop I would stop?
And end it once and for all.
I hate worrying about things that I know won't happen,
But my mind has answered a call
To keep paranoid and stressed out,
Worrying all of my life,
It makes me want to go into a shop
And buy a 10-inch carving knife,
And ram it straight through my diseased mind,
And kill the paranoia inside,
Then pull the knife out and burn it in fire,
And leave the paranoia with nowhere to hide.

THE MINDSET OF A MENTAL PATIENT

But of course, that is not possible.
My mind has a mind of its own.
I beg and plead with it to set me free,
But it won't even give me free time on loan.

Suicide

Yes, I think of suicide,
On a very regular basis.
Yes, I think of suicide,
As a release to permanent stasis.
Yes, I think of suicide,
At the whim of the devilly prancer,
Who would like to make me believe right now
That it would be a life enhancer.

This last poem sums up how I sometimes felt in
2004, and whilst I was feeling dreadful, my poems
gave a little release from the drudgery of work. I
just seemed to be able to come up with rhymes,
and on my breaks each day, I would try to
remember them and commit them to paper. At
this time, paranoia was the centre of my life, and I
wrote the next two poems, the first as my life story
(as an adult) up to this point, and the second
about how paranoia had, since the start of 2004
broken into my life more than ever.

1998 and a Misfiring Brain

1998 and a misfiring brain
Made sure that my life would never be the same,

When Bristol-bound for 3 years I had to travel,
In order to study business psychobabble.

The stresses and strains of moving away
Turned by brain upside down,
And tricks it did play.
There were people out there
Who helped me get through,
But there were less pleasant ones
At the front of the queue,
Who when they heard of the problems I mumbled
Decided that my life was totally bungled.

In the last year, an angel helped me keep semi-
fresh,
I hope to meet him soon,
Again in the flesh,
For with his help I did finally succeed,
But once again, his help I very much need.

The Permanence of Paranoia

Life would be so much simpler if I was dead,
Just like a life permanently confined to my bed.
No worry and no paranoia all of the time,
And a life free of personal fear and crime.

I wonder why I want to live life at all,
And if suicide didn't mean Hell, I'd happily fall.

Some might say I'm just too lazy to live life.
But what's the point of all this terminal trouble and
strife?

THE MINDSET OF A MENTAL PATIENT

It's the permanence of paranoia.
Just the permanence of paranoia.

It's affecting me now at a very big rate,
And my life is trapped inside this confused state.
For so many years, my life has been this way,
And August 1998 was my last happy day.

If suicide didn't mean Hell, I'd happily fall.
Am I waiting here everyday
Just hoping for God's call.
The paranoia of my actions each day
Always just makes it just so hard to cope.
Is my life destined to be that of a Christian without
hope?

This last verse summed up my mental state at the
time. You have probably heard people who have
said that they have gone through periods where
they prayers were just not being answered, and
for me this appeared one of those periods. I
seemed to be stumbling in the darkness, and no
one would turn on the light. The only conclusion I
could come to was that God was punishing me for
something, possibly my blasphemy whilst I had
been at university.

I wanted to die. Several months had passed since
the 9th of January, and anyone else who had
suffered the incident that I had been involved with
would have, quite understandably, put it behind
them and got on with their life, but my brain would

not let me do that. It kept my mental state cold and dark. Just occasionally, it would look like things would get better; those occasions would always be false dawns. My paranoia would notice and get to work to ensure that every time, without fail, that the rug was pulled from under my feet and I would just feel let down and bitter that my mind was clearly not on my side. I suddenly realised one day that since my problems started back in 1998, I had become:

A Prisoner of my Mind

Although I can see clearly,
I am forever blind,
As I struggle through this life of black,
A prisoner of my mind.

It teases, taunts and keeps me,
On a mental ragged edge,
As it entices me invitingly
To that 15th – storey ledge.

"Come on", it says invitingly,
"Let's give gravity a test.
You never know, it might just lead,
To the land of eternal rest."

In know my mind is lying,
For that's the last place it will lead,
As it gorges on my paranoia,
A feast on which to feed.

THE MINDSET OF A MENTAL PATIENT

False Dawns

I thought things were getting better,
But oh, I was so wrong.
It was just another in a series
Of cruel false dawns.
I've been experiencing for so long.

I pray for God to help me,
But get another kick in the teeth,
Which just leaves me down and feeling bitter,
As again, I come to grief.

Will there be a bad outcome this time?
I know there never was before,
But this time it could be different,
As I hurtle back down at break-neck speed
To hit my emotional floor.

Give me a door God,
Give me a way out God,
Kill me and take me away,
Instead of punishing me day in and day out
On an earth on which I don't want to stay.

For whatever I've done wrong God, I'm sorry.
I didn't mean any harm.
Please say you are satisfied now God,
And take me out of this life of alarm.

I've suffered for long enough now God,
For whatever crime I've committed,
But still your punishment rains down on me God,

Tell me, why is it still permitted?

You know I cannot be perfect, God,
As I know is your plan.
I beg you; don't punish me, as I can't God,
Please help me so I can.

This last poem summed up the bitterness I was feeling at this time. I believed that God was punishing me, but He wouldn't confirm why. I would pray to him regularly, begging his assistance to help get me through those troubled times, but (at the time) I thought nothing was happening. I would just keep ending up in situations, which my paranoia would convince me that I would soon be done for. At this time in my life, my brain was very active, but down all of the wrong avenues. Every time something happened to me that left me scared or paranoid, my brain would leap into action, computing all of the conclusions it could think of to the scenarios I was in, each as terrible and improbable as the last, but in my confused state, they all appeared all the more real, just as this next poem describes:

Bottlenecks

At school I was often bullied,
And thought of as a jerk.
In adult life I was issued
With a brain that doesn't work.

The bottlenecks of worrying

THE MINDSET OF A MENTAL PATIENT

Are always, always there.
When one worry's gone,
Another starts,
A break from it is rare.

The devil's plaything is my mind,
Satan's eternal feast?
Or is it God who punishes me?
Have I the mark of the beast?

Whatever it is does its utmost
To make my life a living hell.
The conveyer belt of my worries
Ensure all's never well.

My brain fires off infinite scenarios,
Every single day,
About what the conclusion
To my worries might be,
So I can't find the way.

I can see the correct path to go down,
But my brain won't let me take it,
For though I try,
The worries remain,
I think I'll never make it.

For in this life I've upset God,
So hell in Hell will follow,
After I've finished this hell of life.
There will be no tomorrow.

The last verse is how I felt at the time. I was

feeling so dreadful I was thinking that I must have done something to upset God, and my thoughts returned to the Holy Spirit. Was God punishing me because of what I have done back in 1998? I had managed to get over the problem of thinking of the Holy Spirit all the time some years previously, but was God still not satisfied? It certainly seemed that way. My paranoia was keeping my life black every single day. The only time I could get release was when I was asleep and it could not get to me.

When you are in that situation, imagination and dreams become two of your best friends. In those states, there is nothing there to go wrong, nothing to worry you, everything is wonderful and you can do anything that you want to do. On my lunch breaks at work, I would go and sit in my car and just fantasize for half an hour. I could be anything. A top athlete, an actor, a racing driver, anything that would help me escape from the drudgery I was living in. I would sit there talking to myself, as if I was being interviewed about something I had achieved. My release was…

My Imagination

Nothing is impossible.
Nothing is sad.
Nothing there to torment me
Or make me feel bad,
In my imagination.

THE MINDSET OF A MENTAL PATIENT

Imagination is freedom.
It is the key to my release,
Where for a short time
I can find some sort of mental peace.

If talking to yourself means madness,
I went mad long ago,
To escape from all of my mental problems
That I must overthrow.
Not of imagination.

Imagination is the stuff of dreams,
Where all the good things are,
And all the negative paranoia
Is always so afar.

There I can see long gone loved ones,
And not worry about a thing,
And all of the golden joy bells
Can forever ring.

But it's just my imagination.

Imagination was one of the best parts of my life,
but dreaming was even better, where I could sleep
(which was my favorite activity) and escape from
life at the same time. There was one dream in
particular that I would have regularly, and it was
my favourite one. In it, all of a sudden I would be
able to fly like a bird, with no effort whatsoever. I
could travel hundreds of feet up, and I would
never be scared that I would fall to the ground. In
this dream I would always wish that I was on the

verge of dying and that I could somehow leave earth forever and be accepted into Heaven.

Flying in Dreams

My life is almost over,
At least that's the way it seems.
I really wish it were that way,
When I'm flying in dreams.

It's the only one that re-occurs,
And I fly up so high.
I really wish it were for real,
I want to meet God in the sky.

Every time I dream it,
I pray I'll meet God in Heaven.
I really wish it would come true,
I might just make cloud number seven.

But every time I dream this dream,
I hit the same glass ceiling.
I wish that that part would not happen
In my fantastic dreaming.

It's nice to have a little release,
Although it's sometimes short,
But I really wish it were for real,
And not an incomatose thought.

One day perhaps it will come true,
I'd be with my God Divine,
And I really wish it would come true

THE MINDSET OF A MENTAL PATIENT

That He would take me to Cloud Nine.

Of course, that never happened, and my alarm
clock would ring at every 7am, signaling the end of
my freedom, as these next two poems
demonstrate:

The Dead of Night; the Dread of Day

As I awake in the dead of night,
It's 2.30 AM,
Everything's alright.
No worries or problems to cloud my mind,
The stillness is perfect, I find.

But then comes 7 AM,
The dread of day,
As always, I must find a way,
To overcome my problems
That my brain throws to me.
Its hopelessness it throws right through me.

Just one letter,
The R is the curse,
It drives my life from better to worse.
Is it pre-ordained that my life's this way?
Forever afraid in the dread of day.

It can turn on a sixpence
From minute to minute.
When my life's like this,
My heart's not in it.
Is it the devil, or is it the Lord?

I only know it's punishment,
Of that I'm assured.

I don't know who's my mind's employer,
But I ask God to free me from this paranoia.
He tries, but not in the way, I want.
The way it is, I must be blunt,
Is to punish me from my wavers from love,
The message is clear from the above,
That unless I can fight this one on my own,
Whilst He's always there,
He'll leave me alone.

Since 1998, I have been a fan of Orchestral
Manoeuvres in he Dark, and this poem was
inspired by the piano-melody of their song 'Of All
the Things we've made'.

Bitter Lullaby

Climb in your bed now,
Sleep to the morn,
Your troubles return
At the first light of dawn.

In sleep you'll find freedom,
Some sort of release.
It's the closest you'll ever come
To permanent peace.

Dreaming is heaven,
It's in a place of strife,
Which tears down every single

THE MINDSET OF A MENTAL PATIENT

Part of your life.

Enjoy it while it lasts,
For it will soon go,
And when your eyes open
You'll rejoin your low.

For life is the enemy,
Through birth, now and death.
It will work against you
Till your final breath.

The best part of life's
When you're incomatose,
When you see the beauty,
But no thorns on the rose.

It was at this point in my life that I realized that there was no real point to my existence. My life consisted of going into work each day, trying not to make mistakes in my work, living in constant fear that I was offending people an that I was in danger of losing my job, and then going home on Friday night, fretting about what Monday would bring when I had to return to work. I realized that I was simply…

Going Through the Motions of Life

We're all just going through the motions of life.
Find a job,
Find a wife,
Stay out of trouble,

Christopher J. Fairweather

Always try,
Then make plans for when you die.

I can't believe this is all there is.
There must be more to the plan of His.
But we're all so blind
That we cannot see,
In this world
The great design of He,
Goes unnoticed as we climb the tree.
You get to the top for a sky-high fee.

The branches break when the weight's too great,
When your 35
It's left too late.
If you get into trouble,
You'll feel the pain.
The motions of life will drive you insane.

Complications,
Machinations,
We've reached the culture of compensations.
We all gulp down what's unimportant,
Celebrity culture,
Is this some portent?
Of the punishment for decadence that has now
come.
To what's important, our brains are numb.

Another way is what I seek,
The way of which
I want Him to speak,
Of an alternative

THE MINDSET OF A MENTAL PATIENT

To the motions of life,
Find some meaning
Without the strife.

I do not know the way I seek,
And I know many feel.
That I am some freak,
But when God shows me the way to go,
It will be the correct way, I know.
Anyone who wants to come,
Will be welcome,
They'll be my chum,
For whilst I'm not special,
I'd love to see,
The world turn from its motions.
And come with me.

As this poem suggests, I was going through a phase that many of us go through, that phase being, 'There must be more to life than this,' but I did not know what. All I knew was that my life was mundane and frightening. Mundane in the job I was doing, and frightening because my paranoia would constantly construct scenarios about how I was going to get into trouble, whilst none of these scenarios every actually happened, they all seemed so real. My life was one of regret. Regret that I had ever been born. I felt that I had nothing to offer the world, and that it had nothing to offer me. At this stage, I heard a celebrity, (I cannot remember who) saying that they had no regrets. At the time I never understood people who say this. I thought "How can you go through 85 years on this planet and not regret a single thing that you have done?" I regretted doing things almost every day, such as moving into the house in Bristol that I was thrown out of, the incident, which had started all of my troubles at work. In the depressed state that I was in, I wrote the following poem, about regrets and how I believed they affect all of us:

No one has No Regrets

I want to put it on record,
No one has no regrets.
You can't go through your entire life
Not being upset by all the upsets.
All the wrong decisions made
And all the wrong words said.
You can't not regret them
But only forget them
For a few hours each night in bed.

They're as black as night on the brightest day,
All the mistakes you've made.
All dark in tone,
They won't leave you alone,
As on your mind, they prey.

How could life have turned out,
Had you not gone wrong?
Regrets just automatically occur
And stay with you for so long.

Regrets will ruin everything,

THE MINDSET OF A MENTAL PATIENT

Through life,
Through death,
Through besets,

So now, I am finally putting it on record,
NO ONE HAS NO REGRETS.

It was also at this point that I wrote the poem that a few years later would lead my psychiatrist to suggest the possibility of Asperger's Syndrome to me. This poem is about a subject, which had been in my mind for some years. I had often felt somewhat distant from the people around me, whether it had been at school, university or the work place. When I was walking down a street in a town, although people would be walking close to me, I felt separated from them as if I was a stranger in a foreign land. This led to me writing a poem, which whilst it seems a little naïve now is about something, which I had thought about for a number of years, before and after my problems really started:

Am I an Alien?

I could be an alien
Who's come from outer space,
At least that's the way I feel,
Living amongst the human race.

I feel like an outsider,
With brain programming gone wrong,
Misfiring and jumping from its groove

Into a different song.

Somehow, I feel different,
And not one of the crowd,
But my alien race won't tell me for certain.
They will not lift the shroud.

I don't know if I'm one of us,
Or if I'm one of them.
I wish I could go back to my home planet
And start my life again.
Am I here to tell this other race
Of what life on earth is like?
Surely they've seen enough by now
To let me take a hike,
Back to the space from which I've come,
To start my life once more,
Before the life I live on earth
Brings me mentally to the floor.

It was at this point that I decided that I needed to
get some extra medical assistance. I would see
my GP and psychiatrist at regular intervals to
discuss how things were going, but I was feeling
very vulnerable.

Most of the people I worked with were women,
and by this time I was so scared of upsetting any
of them, I must admit I did behave rather strangely
at times. One of my jobs was to regularly take
packages from my office down to the post room,
and as time passed and I started to take longer
routes to get the post room, simply because I

knew I would meet fewer people on the route, and hence give my brain fewer causes to fire off its paranoid thoughts that scared me.

After discussing with my GP and psychiatrist, it was agreed that I would be offered another Community Nurse to help with the problems that I was having.

I felt that having the extra support would be helpful to me, and so it was. The nurse I had this time was a lady called Jo, and she was also invaluable to me. During our first meeting in December 2004, I explained to her all about my troubles, and I ended up on a course of cognitive therapy with her. The first thing that I had to do was to try and face up to the fears I had of offending people, trying to surreptitiously find out if I had offended them, and constantly apologising to people who I thought I had offended when I hadn't, and try to conquer them. I was totally scared at the thought of having to do this, but I realized that there was no other option. It was not going to be easy, and I knew that in the short-term things might get worse as I tried to do without the various safety behaviors that I had adopted since the incident, which had occurred in January. These safety behaviors included glancing away from people every 2-3 seconds when I was talking to them, along with the other three discussed above. But there was no alternative. I knew that if I did not try to conquer them, I would be a slave to them forever, and I did not want that at all. I knew that I should take Jo's advice, knuckle down and pray that God would finally smile on me and help me out of the mental mess that I was in.

CHAPTER FIVE

BEGINNING THE FIGHTBACK

<u>Fightback</u>

What I worry about is nonsense,
And what I worry about's not right,
But from now on my stupid worries,
Won't keep me waking up all night.

It won't be easy,
Of that, I am assured.
I must increase the faith I have
To believe in the Good Lord.

This is the fightback,
It won't be easy
But I've got to get up now.
This is the fightback,
I need to trust in the Good Lord.
To show me how.

I've made me live in darkness,

But now I've turned on the light,
To shine a way out of this blackness,
I now must cease from mental fright.

This is the fightback,
It won't be easy
But I've got to get up now.
This is the fightback,
I need to trust in the Good Lord.
To show me how.

After a couple of appointments with Jo, I wrote this
poem to give myself a beam of hope, and to try
and make myself believe that I could conquer my
problems and that God would help me. I truly
believed then, as I do now that it was a matter of
faith. I had suddenly realised that in a strange
way that God had been keeping me safe, because
whilst it is true that I had been living in a state of
perpetual fear for most of 2004, none of my
worries and fears had come to any fruition, and
with the benefit of hindsight I could see that I had
in fact been worrying about nothing in that respect.
I was still not quite sure why God was letting my
worries happen in the first place however. Often I
would pray to him, asking why he still allowed me
to suffer, but then, after a while I started to see
things in a rather different light. Up to this point I
thought that I had been sent all of my worries as a
punishment, but then I thought that perhaps they
were being sent as a test of my faith, and if this
was the case I certainly did not want to be found

wanting. But just as the poem above says, I knew that it was not going to be easy.

One thing that did help however, was that the girl that I had offended at the start of the year when my problems began, had managed to get herself a better job and was not working in my office anymore so that was one less person I had to worry about offending. But as I have pointed out earlier, my brain worries about the what-ifs, and in doing so my brain was now trying to make me believe that before she left she might have told some other people in the office about what had happened. This meant that up to a point I was still living in fear of offending my colleagues. If one of them happened to pass me in the morning, and say "Good Morning," to me in anything less than a very happy tone of voice, my brain would still turn it into a declaration of war, and even worse, if they passed me and did not say anything at all, the paranoia in my brain would try to convince me that I had definitely upset them. However, I knew that I had to overcome these fears. I could no longer avoid my colleagues and try to talk to them as little as possible. I had to be able to talk to them and not appear afraid. And so I tried. Sometimes I was able to, and I felt a little stronger, but the paranoia was still there, and sometimes in weeks where I could not do a thing without worrying constantly, I felt like rolling over and giving up:

Black and White Rainbows

The fight back comes to nothing,
The Devil sees to that.
I'm left just chasing black and white rainbows.
I'm knocked out on the mat.

I'll probably never make the count,
I'm blinded by the starts,
The devil is going all out now
To make me want to contract SARS.

Death seems like the only way,
To get out of this mental mire.
All my wrongs magnify around me,
My conscience is a liar.

My brain's my biggest enemy,
Of it, the Devil's in control.
He makes my problems seem ten times worse,
As I'm dragged all over the burning coal.

There's no release,
There's no way out,
No more, fight back
I sadly shout.
Just black and white rainbows
And paranoid frowns,
To lock me forever
With tears of clowns.

THE MINDSET OF A MENTAL PATIENT

Life in the Beehive

Stung to death in life's beehive,
And waiting for God at 25.
The wax in the honey
Is so bitter for me,
Should I have ended my life at 23?
The burning in hell would be torture I know,
Of forever and 700 days below.
There's no way I want it,
And though life is a blow,
It is somewhat better than the Devil and co.
I'm paranoid and worried 24/7,
But I hope that this life
Will take me soon up to Heaven.

There's no upside to life
No matter how hard I try,
So the question I ask is just,
My life, why?

This next poem was inspired by the aquarium that
we have in the living room at my house.

A Heavenly Prison

The six-foot glass aquarium
Is a heavenly prison for tropical fish,
And my desire to join them now
Is my one undying wish.

I know that life might be rather dull,
And I wouldn't live that long,

But oh to live a happy short life
Where nothing at all goes wrong.

It's not so great being human,
And I'm a lucky one,
Where life for most is a daily burning,
By the dark side of the sun.

The fish tank water would extinguish
All my deepest fears,
And give me nothing to worry about
For be it months or years.

And finally, with the 3 second memory
That fish apparently know,
Each day would be a new adventure,
And not a tale of woe.

This last poem was written during a particularly dark period of my life, when anything seemed better than being a human. I began to see how whilst some of us have all the material comforts that life can provide, at the same time for some reason in the western world we seem to have the ability to make life as difficult as possible for ourselves, and this inevitably makes life more stressful. It is stress that can trigger mental health conditions such as that which I was suffering from. From the time I had experienced living adult life I could now see why so many people now suffer from some mental health problem. We have just made our lives so darn complicated, and things show no signs of getting better:

THE MINDSET OF A MENTAL PATIENT

Castles in the Sky

As I live my life every day,
I often wonder why,
As I'm happiest when I staying at home
Building castles in the sky.

Of course, up there it's impossible
To get any foundations dug.
I know these dreams will never happen,
But I've been bitten by the bug,
Of creating various perfections
That I know will never be,
But it's my happiest pastime,
I could do it infinitely.

But after time the castle I'm living in
Always disappears,
And I nosedive down to the barren earth,
In my mind there forms salt tears.
For the greatest builders cannot build
A cottage in the sky,
But I'd be happy if they could.
I wish that they would try.

So my dreams are dreams and nothing more,
But comfort they provide,
And form some sort of dwelling
In which from my life I can hide.

It was at this dark time in my life that I started to
take a big interest in the poems of Spike Milligan.
I had been a fan of The Goon Show for years, and

I knew that he had written many books of poems as well. I also knew that he had been a manic-depressive and had spent some periods of his life in institutions where he had written some very dark and serious verse. But I also knew that he had written many very funny poems, particularly his nonsense verse. I thought it very interesting that someone who had periods of life that were as black as his could also write the wonderful nonsense that he did. This set me thinking. By now, I had written a lot of dark poems myself. Obviously, they were not as good as his were, for how could they possibly be? But I began to wonder if I could write funny poems as well. I knew that writing poems about the problems I was suffering often made me feel a little less worried about them, and I was thinking that writing funny poems might help me as well, that is if I could write them. I decided that there was no harm in trying, and that I would try writing a funny poem in the style of Spike Milligan, and below is the result. When all said and done, I am not sure how faithful to Spike's writing style it was, but I was quite pleased with the result:

Inventor Jimmy

Inventor Jimmy is on his toil,
With kitchen scissors and engine oil,
He invented the hybrid motorised Thrun,
Which helps people with unequal legs to run,
So instead of in circles they can now run straight,
But in winter only until it's half past eight,

THE MINDSET OF A MENTAL PATIENT

For sadly the device is solar powered,
(So of course, it's no use to Michael Howard).

But he's planning a version that will work in the
dark,
So they can run from King's Cross to Regent's
Park,
And catch the performance of Elsie Thrigg,
Who's inventing the inflatable oil rig,
Which is of course is needed to supply all the oil
For the Mark II Thrun's essential coil,
And when it's invented then all will be free,
To run in straight lines quite easily.

Feeling a little buoyed up by the result, and
realising that I could also write other types of
poem, I managed to write the following poem,
which is a true story about my early days at
university. I had had the basic idea for this poem
for a while, but it was only now that I was able to
find the inspiration and the ideas to write the
finished article, and for anyone who is going away
to university for the first time, here is a chance to
learn from my mistakes!

The Perils of Powdered Milk

Powdered Milk tastes horrible,
Of that, I guarantee.
The taste is quite intolerable,
So stick to UHT!

The only time I tried it

Was in 1998,
I poured it on my cereal,
(Which I ate at a slow rate),
So fresh milk was not practical,
As quickly it went off,
And gave a horrible flavour
To the flakes I tried to scoff.
So after much deep thinking, I thought,
"I know what I'll do,
I'll buy a tin of powdered milk,
For cereal and tea too!"

So off I went to Tesco
And bought the biggest I could find.
I thought this would be the answer,
How could I be so blind?
I got this tin of stuff back home
And thought, "How much shall I make,
To pour all over my cereal,
And to cover every flake?"

But when I looked at the conversion chart,
My troubles had begun.
It didn't go low enough for three bowls of flakes,
Let alone just one!

So I got the calculator out and
And found the ratio.
I poured the milk over the flakes,
Took a spoon and thought, "here we go!"

But the resulting mixture was disgusting,
So here's the advice for all to see:

THE MINDSET OF A MENTAL PATIENT

Powdered milk tastes horrible,
So stick to UHT!

I was very happy that I was able to write
something which I found amusing, even if no-one
else did, and I found writing them a very
therapeutic way of helping to distract my mind of
all the worries that my paranoia tried to overpower
me with. I was feeling a little better about myself,
until something happened one day at work, which
led to writing another type of poem, and one,
which at the time chilled me to the core. It was a
Friday at work and I was going about my business
when suddenly I heard that my two managers had
been called away to a hastily conceived and
urgent meeting. As it always did at times like this,
my paranoia sprung into action and my brain went
into overdrive. Had this meeting been called
because of something I had done? Was I in
trouble? Whilst my common sense tried to keep
me worry free, my brain and paranoia were having
none of it, I felt scared and physically sick. On my
lunch break that day, I sat in my car and wrote
this:

The Agony (circa 2005)

The paranoia is agony.
Is this meeting to do with me?
Have I done something wrong?
Every time something unexpected happens
I am filled with a cold agony
Which will last forever,

Until the result comes through.
My mind trawls through all the mistakes I might
have made,
But I don't know if I have.
The agony constricts my brain,
Like a snake squeezing the breath out of its prey,
The agony squeezes the hope out of my mind,
And replaces it with paranoia and dread.
Will the whole weekend be like this
Before I am killed on Monday morn?
Or is all this just coincidence,
Like it normally is?

But the agony will not let go.
"It might be different this time," it says,
Like it always says.
It's vice like grip controls all of me.
The balance of probability means nothing to it.
"If it could happen it will" is its maxim.

It will be like this until I know the answer.
I know not when that will be,
Or if I will survive this time.

The agony looks ahead to the nigh-on,
Sixty years it has controlling me,
Unless the Devil gets me first.
I'm sure they work together,
Battling against God for control of me.
It will be like this forever.

Please God, take me from here to you,
End my life for me,

THE MINDSET OF A MENTAL PATIENT

And make it right for me in Heaven.
Amen.

It was another of those moments I sometimes had in my life when life seemed hopeless and pointless and that there was no point to my existence, but what I did not know then was that soon, through an unpleasant experience at work I was able to see the possibility of a new dawn.

Christopher J. Fairweather

CHAPTER SIX

A NEW DAWN?

2005 was the year when it suddenly became apparent to the management of the company I worked for was not as good as it should have been. One day we were all called into a staff meeting and were told the news. There was to be a recruitment freeze and any staff leaving the department would not be replaced. We were also told that there would be the threat of redundancies. Also all the agency staff would be lost immediately.

At the same time, the distinct impression was given that the top management of the organisation were expecting us to carry on providing a full-strength service without the necessary resources. As you can imagine, morale plummeted.

Just prior to this happening, I had been looking in the recruitment section of my local paper and had seen that an academic library quite close to where I lived was advertising for an overall Library Manager on a very good salary. I thought that I probably did not have the qualifications that they were looking for, but I would get an application pack anyway to see what it was all about. When it arrived, it was as I suspected. The qualification they were asking for was a post-graduate one in Library Management, which I did not have, but the thought crossed my mind about finding out which universities offered such as qualification. I was to find out much sooner than I had anticipated.

As the weeks went by at work, morale did not improve and cutbacks became more likely. I was working all hours just to keep my area on an even keel, and several people were complaining that we were not keeping up with the work, and had little sympathy for our staff and resource shortages. One day, after a particularly difficult and fraught morning, I decided that I had had enough. I wanted out and soon. So I decided to find out about universities that offered courses in library management. I telephoned Learn Direct and to cut a long story short, I ended up applying for an MA in Information and Library Management at Loughborough University. As the weeks went by and I waited for a reply from the university, I was quite tense. I so wanted to get out of where I was, but I wanted to be doing something more fulfilling than stacking shelves at Tesco again.
Finally, I received a call inviting me for an interview at Loughborough University, which I

went to. Before I even visited the campus, I was impressed with university. Obviously, when I applied to them I had to fill in the medical questionnaire, which I have always been suspicious of. I declared my mental health problems, fearing this would count against me, as I believed it had done on many jobs I had applied for, but there was no need for me to worry. Shortly after I sent the form off, I received a letter from a man who I would get to know well.He was in charge of ensuring that people with mental health problems who were on the campus were cared for. In his letter, he was offering to help me with various things, including applying for assistance that students with disabilities are entitled to. I was very impressed by this. Visiting the university campus was also quite an experience. When I had first visited the University of the West of England in Bristol, where I had done my first degree, I had felt like a stranger in a foreign land, and it was unnerving. But Loughborough was different. It seemed friendlier and less intimidating, even though I was nervous about the interview.

I arrived at the Department of Information Science where the interview was going to take place. I was met by one of senior lecturers who would interview me. She was very friendly. We talked about why I had applied. She asked me some questions, and at the end said, she was going to offer me an unconditional place for the coming academic year. I was overjoyed. Finally, perhaps things were going to improve for me. I left the department with my mind in whirl. I had had no idea that I would be offered a place on the same day as the interview. Then I had an idea. I had my mobile phone with me, so I telephoned the Mental Health Officer and explained that I had just been offered a place for the new academic year, and whilst I would understand if he was too busy to see me (as I did not have a prior appointment to him), did he have any time free? He agreed to see me. I went to his office and we had a conversation about my mental problems, and he was very understanding about them. He told me about the help that was on offer, and what he could do for me, including a regular meeting with one of his colleagues who was a counsellor. Next, I asked him about how I should go about finding accommodation in Loughborough, explaining the bad experience I had had in Bristol. Again, help was at hand. He explained that he had a small number of accommodation places reserved for people with disabilities and mental health problems, and one of them was a small studio flat just across the road from the campus. Things just kept getting better! He explained to me that he could hold it for me for a few days whilst I thought everything over.

I returned home that day on the train with my mind buzzing. My experience had been a contrast to my experiences in Bristol, where whilst I must stress they had been sympathetic about my problems once they had started, (and had granted

THE MINDSET OF A MENTAL PATIENT

me uncapped referrals if I had needed to retake any exams), but I had not experienced as much assistance as I had experienced at Loughborough, and this was after one day!

Over the next few days, I decided that I would take up the offer of the University place, and the studio flat that was being held for me. Finally, everything seemed to be falling into place for me after a long and uncertain period of waiting.

Shortly after this, I gave my notice at work. I was very glad to be going. I knew that I would miss the people but not the job. My managers had been most understanding about the mental health problems that I had, and whilst I had been scared of offending my colleagues in the office where I worked, none of them had ever complained about me and they had usually been nice to me, as always it was my brain constructing problems that did not exist, but overall I was still glad to be going. On my last day I was presented with a card, which had so many good wishes from people in it, I realised that it was indeed my brain that was not on my side, and that it was the people at work who were. They are too numerous to mention here, but I would like to thank them all for putting up with me and being accepting of me with my condition, which is far more than certain other people in the past had been.

On Friday September 30th 2005 I loaded up my car, said goodbye to my family and set off for

Loughborough. The journey was uneventful and I arrived in the late afternoon where I was given my key card so I could get access to my flat, which was in a building in the Halls of Residence where many other students lived. I arrived at my flat, which was on the top floor. It was quite small, but it had everything I needed, and I liked it. Over the evening, I brought all my things up to my flat and got settled for the night.

The following day I went into the town, and I liked what I saw. It had everything. Shops of all varieties, several banks, a good supermarket and convenient bus stops. I bought some items of stationary and returned home, feeling very happy.

My first month on the campus passed happily and reasonably uneventfully. I rapidly established a small circle of friends who I got on with, and things looked good. The only downside was that my fear of offending people was still there, and there were some people on my course who seemed (to my paranoid brain) to be a little less friendly and my brain tried to make me think that I had offended them like it had done so many times before, but it was all still much better than my experiences in Bristol.

Soon, I met my new GP, who was at a practice based on the campus, and the counsellor who I had been told about, and both of them were very good at helping me with the worries I was having.

THE MINDSET OF A MENTAL PATIENT

For sometime, I did not feel the need to write as many poems as I had been doing. Normally I felt the need to write poems about my mental health only when I was going through periods of serious worry, and at the time I was not. But, I was inspired to try and keep writing funny poems, again just to see if I could. Also, after seeing a poster somewhere on the campus about mental health problems, I got the inspiration to write the following poem. It was partly based on personal experience, and also echoed the advertising style of the poster:

Labels

I'm a tin in the corner shop of life,
You'll find me on a shelf,
For people always pass me by,
Despite their material wealth.

They pick me up and look at me,
And read my label now and then,
But then they pull a disgusted face,
And put me down again.

For so long they had done this,
And I really didn't know why.
I knew soon I'd pass my sell-by date,
And then the end would be nigh.

So one day I gave my plight some thought,
And wondered, "How am I labeled?"
Then a man picked me up and said to his mate,

Christopher J. Fairweather

"Look, this tin says disabled."

So he put me down
And they hurried away,
And at last, the truth was clear.
It was the way I was labeled
That had sealed by fate,
Day after month after year.

So if you see me in life's corner shop,
Pick me up for I won't hurt you.
I might say disabled on my outside,
But on the inside, I have virtue.

So I'll end by telling you all right now,
As I sit next to life's Black Treacle,
Please keep an open mind,
And do not be unkind,
For labels are for cans not people.

This poem was based upon the strapline of the advert, which is also the last line of the above poem.

Also, around this time I finally got the inspiration to write another silly poem about a subject that had been on my mind since I was 4 years old. When I was young, my mother would often give me Marmite on toast, which I quite liked. However, I always found the Marmite rather strong, and one day when was young and looking through the larder at home, I found another jar, which was exactly the same shape as a Marmite, jar. It also had a black substance inside. Of course, it was Bovril, and one day I asked my mother if I could try Bovril on toast instead. She agreed, and I have never eaten Marmite since!

Ambivalent About Marmite

Ambivalent about Marmite
Is a strange thing to be,
As most either love it
Or hate it you see.
If spread too thickly
It tastes far too strong,
And is far too powerful
For a gum to take on,
As it penetrates the lining
Surrounding your teeth,
You feel it biting into
Your enamel beneath.
But if spread quite thinly
It can taste quite nice,
But not as nice as Bovril,
Which I'd choose in a trice.
I know Bovril on toast
It can seem quite odd,
But in Bovril versus Marmite,
I'd give Bovril the nod,
As Bovril's not quite as strong
I have found, you see,
So when I'm eating my toast
It's Bovril for me.
So if ambivalent about Marmite,
Give Bovril a try.

You might find it nicer,
And that is no lie.

Later that year, in December, I would meet a
woman who would in some ways change my life.
She was my new Psychiatrist . The first time I
went to see her, I gave a copy of the poems I had
written so she could a get as good idea as
possible about how my mental problems had
affected me. For a long time I have believed that I
was able to articulate how I felt about myself
through writing poems better than just telling
someone in normal speech, even though when
you are talking normally you have the entire
language at your disposal and are not restricted to
words that have to rhyme and scan with each
other. As it was to turn out, I am very glad that I
did show her my poems, including one, which I
had written shortly before I met her for the first
time. Whilst it is similar to a poem mentioned
earlier in this book (Am I an Alien?) it summed up
an experience I had in December, and it finally
gave the inspiration to write a poem about how I
felt on this occasion, and had often felt at times
going right back to when I was young. On this
occasion I had gone, on a Saturday to see Harry
Potter and the Goblet of Fire. When I emerged
from the cinema, it was dark, and as I walked
through the people who were in the town
shopping, I came up with the words of this poem:

THE MINDSET OF A MENTAL PATIENT

The Distant Visitor

The distant visitor
Is a distant prisoner,
For all of his time upon earth.
This distant visitor
Is a distant prisoner,
Until the time of his death
From the moment of birth.

Human life is what's distant,
And the distance persistent,
Through night and through day
And through time.
Though just a few feet away
Far from me they stay,
And I cannot cross over their line.

So I'm a distant observer,
An alien receptor,
Feeding on life upon earth.
For whilst I'm not in it
I move along with it,
Until the time of my death,
But not with much mirth.

For my home is so distant
And my people resistant,
To my pleas to be brought back to home.
So until they do it,
On earth I'll go through it,
Seeing life with my tired fine-toothed comb.

It was this poem (along with others) that my psychiatrist to suggest to me (at our first meeting in 2006) that I might have a condition called Asperger's Syndrome. As I have said earlier, Asperger's Syndrome has been talked about by some as a person having 'a dash of Autism.' Like Autism, and mental health problems as a whole, the spectrum of its severity is broad and wide, but in general, its problems can include the sufferer finding it difficult to interact with others and lacking certain social skills. When I was told this, it struck a chord with me. As I have said earlier, ever since I was young, I had always felt that I did not really fit in with many of the other pupils at the schools I went to. I had always been a loner, with few friends, and I had often been teased and taunted by other pupils for being a bit strange and a little different. This led me to keep myself to myself as much as possible, and often when I had gone to friends' birthday parties, I had often felt like a fish out of water, but I never quite knew why. I was also told that the minds of people with Asperger's Syndrome are often different. Sometimes they have an obsession with one subject for no particular reason. This was definitely true with me. From a very young age, I had been fascinated by cars. You might very understandably say that there is nothing strange about this, but my fascination went further. My Mother tells me that by the time I was 2 years old, I could walk down the street with her in the town where we lived and name the make and model of *every* car at the side of the road.

THE MINDSET OF A MENTAL PATIENT

At the time, no one had thought much about this. Asperger's Syndrome was not a recognised condition until 1993, and whilst it might have seemed a little strange, it was not a serious problem. When I was five or six, a similar thing happened with me and mazes. I had never heard of them or knew what they were until I was watching an episode of Record Breakers one afternoon. They were visiting the hedge maze at Longleat, which is the largest of its type in the world. All of a sudden, I was fascinated with mazes, as I still am to this day.

When I told my psychiatrist this, it seemed to suggest that perhaps Asperger's Syndrome was indeed what I had, and it certainly answered a lot of questions for me about why I was how I was. Therefore, I was able to go forward feel more relaxed about myself. Unfortunately this happy state of affairs was not to last long, as in the new year, thanks to a record I listened to, I was about to come down with a new mental health problem, which was one that would cause me a lot of heartache and worry.

Christopher J. Fairweather

CHAPTER SEVEN

O
C
D

The three letters O.C.D. were soon to rule my life. They stand for Obsessive Compulsive Disorder. How I came to acquire an Obsessive Compulsive Disorder is a strange story. For a while, before I went away to university in Loughborough I had become a fan of the satirical songs of the American entertainer Tom Lehrer. In this country, he is probably best known for his comedy song called Poisoning Pigeons in the Park, which is a very funny song about that particular activity, and this was the song that attracted me to his work. Over time, I collected a boxed set of his work, which included a song called National Brotherhood Week, which was a satirical song about sections of US society and how they reacted to towards others in 1960s America, e.g. the racial struggles of black people and how people of one faith acted towards another. The song is not at all racist; it merely paints a satirical picture of what 1960s America was like. I found the song was funny, whilst it was making a valid point at the same time.

As with many songs that I like, I would sometimes have it on playback in my head, and there was no problem with this to begin with, but that would change after I bought another record at a record fair in November 2005. In additional to liking satirical songs I also liked songs, which had totally silly lyrics, and this was how I came to buy a copy of a song made by the ITV team who had made the programme Spitting Image in the 1980s/90s. The 'A' Side was a mickey take of the silly holiday songs, which groups such as Black Lace would often release, and this was the reason I bought it. However, it was the 'B' Side that was to be the start of my problems. It was called 'I've never met a Nice South African.' It must be pointed out that when this song was originally released in 1986, South Africa was still very much under the grip of dreadful apartheid, and Nelson Mandela was still in prison. The song was very funny and was poking fun at the racists who believed that they were superior simply because they were white.

I listened to the song and some of the words remained in my head.

Some weeks later, I was in one of the washrooms in the library at Loughborough University, and I happened to be thinking about the lyrics of this song, and those of National Brotherhood Week, when from inside my cubicle I heard another person washing their hands, and suddenly I was struck with fear. For the life of me, I could not remember if I had just been thinking about the lyrics, or if I had actually been singing them quietly to myself. The university campus was very much multi-racial, and as it always did in situations like this, my paranoid brain rushed in all directions, trying to convince me that if the person had been black, or of one of the ethnic groups mentioned in the songs, and had heard anything I might have been singing, they might very understandably be offended, and complain about me. This led me back to all the fears I had about offending people, getting into trouble and being sacked, except as I was at university, I feared being expelled instead.

Rather shaken and frightened I emerged from my cubicle. The other person in the washroom had gone. I stepped out of the washroom and into the library, standing in the queue at the issue desk were a group of oriental students. I suddenly got the terrible fear that I was about to blurt some horrible racist insult such at them. Words were dancing around my brain, taunting me. My paranoia went into overdrive, trying to convince me that I had said something, when I didn't think I had. In panic, I fled from the library, and began to walk home. It was the middle of the afternoon and people of all ethnic origins were going about their business on the campus. I was so scared. I managed to get home, in a frightened state, with horrible racist insults racing around my brain, begging my mouth to utter them and cause offence and anger to others who had done nothing to me.

A few days passed, and the problem resolutely refused to go away. I made an appointment to see my doctor about this new problem. I figured that if I did this, and then I accidentally uttered some abhorrent insult by accident I could at least say I had spoken to my doctor about it, that I was ashamed of it and had not wanted to do it on purpose. Shortly after this, I told my counsellor on the campus, and when I my psychaitrist, I told her as well. It was she who believed it was Obsessive Compulsive Disorder, and gave me a few strategies to try and help it, such as wearing a rubber band on my wrist and twanging it against my wrist when I feared saying something wrong, thus distracting myself. She also told me to try to relax if I feared saying something wrong.

I found that trying to relax helped me a little, the problem was that I sometimes forgot to try and relax, as I was so consumed by the thought of offending someone and my paranoia would still always try and convince me that I had said something, The other problem that I had was that one of my friends on the campus was quite openly gay, and soon I was scared that I might spout insults towards him as well as people of other races. I would end up talking to him at times and later on going back to him just to check I hadn't offended him at all, which I don't doubt he found rather strange when he did not know why I was asking.

This new problem was also making life outside of the university difficult as well. Loughborough is a multi-ethic town, and many of the residents were black, and trying to interact normally was now much more difficult. I must stress that I am not a racist and I deplore racism in all its forms, but every time I got on a bus I was scared of offending the driver (if they happened to be black) when I was buying my ticket, and then he might complain to the police, who then might arrest me for saying horrid racist things.

Once again, I felt very depressed, scared and alone. This reminded of an uncle I had who had died just over a year earlier. He had been a bachelor all of his life, and in his later years he became depressed and maudlin. It was widely felt by my family that he too had mental health problems, but unlike me he refused to take medication, which made his problems even worse. It had often been said that I took after my Uncle John, and in my depressed state, I started to wonder if I would end up like him:

Uncle John and the Eternal Dilemma

My Uncle John was a lonely man,
When his spirit escaped his body and ran.
He died friendless and he died alone,
Inside his crumbling Caister home.

Christopher J. Fairweather

His brain was misfiring (just like mine),
And so it was a release when God called time,
But thanks to my brain and it's evil scheming,
In his footsteps I'm dragged kicking and
screaming.

In future will I sit alone in my house?
My only company being a haggard woodlouse,
For with other people I find it hard to interact,
And that's not a sob story that is a fact.

For in my brain, my paranoia's a marauder,
That and my Obsessive Compulsive disorder,
This gives me the fear that I will say
Offensive things to others every single day.
Which will cause me to offend,
And my freedom to cease,
When someone who subsequently calls the police,
Thinks I'm a racist or a homophobic man,
And thought I wanted to offend when it wasn't my
plan.

So, afraid of others and my paranoia's stealth,
My spirit has had cause to turn in on itself,
And I try to hide from others, who I think I might
curse,
Though I know this will just affect my life for the
worse.

So it's tough to make friends,
But if I stay alone,
I'll be Uncle John Junior with a life dark in tone,

THE MINDSET OF A MENTAL PATIENT

Living life scared and friendless
And alone just like him.
When I think of it like that
The future looks very dim.

If I go on like this my next celebration,
Will be from beyond the grave after my cremation,
When I know that my paranoia can no longer get
to me,
After a life where it penetrated and soaked right
through me.

So I look forward to my death and I pray for some
sun,
When my spirit has escaped my body and run,
And I must say that my Uncle John got the last
laugh,
But Dear Lord give me the strength not to follow
his path.

By now, all of the old problems were coming back.
When I spoke to friends or teaching staff on the
campus I would be looking for slightest suggestion
though their body language and the tone of their
voice to try and work out if I had done or said
something to offend them, or if they knew I was
going to be in trouble for anything else that I had
done, and once again, I was feeling the same as I
had done previously.

At times like this, it would have been easy to think
that I was the only one suffering, but I knew that 1
in 4 people in the country will suffer some form of

mental health problem during their lives, many of them more serious than my own, and this knowledge in a strange way comforted me. One night I was watching Bremner, Bird and Fortune on Channel 4, and John Fortune happened to utter the first line of what inspired me to write this next poem:

Stigmatised

On and on and on and on,
Without any rhyme or reason.
On and on and on and on,
No matter what the season.
Down and down and down and down
Through the black we hurtle,
And round and round and round and round
We travel in an endless circle.

With mental illness
There is no sun,
But there is a stigma
For all and for one,
Who suffer and often dare not tell
Any others about their living hell.
For with mental problems
The spectrum is wide,
But the stigma about them
Means that we must hide
Our illness from friends,
Who might just think it naff,
But often sadly think
We're a dangerous psychopath.

THE MINDSET OF A MENTAL PATIENT

That's the stigma we suffer, you see,
And others might think that
(If we told them for free).
We hope they might sympathize,
For better or worse,
But they've heard the lies,
And they heard them first,
That all who suffer
Are all the same,
And that we're all psychos
In all but name,
So if you told them
And things got much worse,
And they didn't sympathize,
That's the curse of the curse.

So on and on and on we go
Without any rhyme or reason.
On and on and on we crawl,
No matter what the season,
And how much better our lives would be,
If only our cause was stronger.
But we are the cursed.
Will death get us first?
I scream "For how much longer?"

Indeed, I did think 'for how much longer?' Again, I
started to wonder if I was being punished. Some
people who believe in reincarnation believe that
we are reincarnated to be punished for the sins of
a previous life. I had never really thought about it
until now, but all of a sudden, it made a lot of

sense. I wondered what terrible crimes I had committed in a previous life to have given what I was living with now, and whilst thinking about this, I concocted the following theories:

Endless Circles

When I signed up for life
What on earth was I doing?
I must have been drunk,
With my reason ungluing.
I must pass life's exam
To get back up to Heaven,
But there's no chance of that,
As my senses, they deaden.
All hope about life
Just does not exist.
I'm just waiting for its end,
And also, it's twist,
For I know something will go wrong,
And I will not win,
And I'll have to live my life
One more time for my sin.

But in that next life
I'll go wrong once again,
And be sent back to earth
With my fellow sinning men.
And next time I come back
I'll miss my old others,
I won't have the friends
I can treat like a brothers.

THE MINDSET OF A MENTAL PATIENT

So next time I'll come back
To the same problems but worse,
And in all my future lives
I will live with this curse.
I'll exist infinitely
With all of this strife.
Oh why on earth,
Did I sign up for life?

Sentenced to Life

I've finally worked out what I'm doing on earth,
I've been sentenced to life.
89 years surrounded by my worst fears,
Yes, I've been sentenced to life.

I don't play its game but it's still all the same,
It happens whether I want it or not.
Being an adult's no fun,
From it I'd like to run.
I wish I was still confined to my cot.

It's true that school days were the best of my life,
But that's not saying too much.
The bullying went on,
That the days would be gone,
Now I'm locked up in adult life's hutch.

I see the world go by but it's all one big lie,
I'm damned within or without.
In or out of the hutch life's just far too much,
With eternal fear and nagging self-doubt.

So I won't play the game,
I will not live life,
I won't test the water,
I won't find a wife.
For the water is boiling,
And my wife she would leave,
So I appeal to the Great One for parole and
reprieve.

As before, I started looking back to the past for
comfort. I had always liked little unimportant
things that I was able to enjoy when I was young.
Back then, I loved adverts on television, and I was
able to find some old videos, which had some of
them on. Other silly things like old ITV idents that
you used to get before an ITV programme such as
Thames, TVS, and LWT etc. I freely admit I look
at the past through totally rose-tinted spectacles,
and I make no apology for it. If David Tennant
arrived in his TARDIS tomorrow, offering to take
me back to spend the week in 1981, I would jump
at the chance. Whilst I also agree that there has
never been a golden age, and that the 1980s was
a bad time for a lot of people, I have an affection
for the time I was growing up in, in the same way
other people would have affection for the 50s and
60s. It was at this time I wrote the following poem.
Whilst it revisits some themes of previous poems
in this book, it also explains how I feel about the
past. It was not all wonderful, but I have the
certainty of knowing that I got through all of life's
trials back then, when I did not know if I would get
through this one now:

THE MINDSET OF A MENTAL PATIENT

A Rose-Tinted Curates Egg

Clinging to the past,
Clinging to the last,
With a rose-tinted view of the past years lived
through.

Imagination and dreams
Are so good it seems,
Of a curate's egg memory with which I make do.

But the bitterness of hindsight
Which greets me a first light,
Lives with me as I stumble though life,
With the people there who bated me,
The people there who hated me,
And teased regularly and ensured it was always
rife.

I know religiously revenge is wrong,
But I have wanted it for far too long,
Against those others who did cause me so much
pain.
If I had reported them,
I know I could have thwarted them,
And thrown back to them some of their rain.

But in spite of all this taunting,
Which at the time I found so daunting,
The past looks better when it's in the past.
I would like to travel back there,
Even though there was a lack there of good times,
But the ones that were there always last.

For there were people there who were nice,
As with others I would dice,
And their sneering and superiority,
For there was my mother's mother,
Who was more than just another,
And I treasure my walks with her by the sea.

It all seems better than today,
I wish there was another way
To enjoy the past and forget about the present,
And relive all the good times
Without all the bad times,
Which I've learnt to hate and now resent.

But a rose-tinted curate's egg is for what I now
beg,
As you can't have the good times without the bad,
Because the certainty of the whole past
Is what with me will last,
Even though that some of it was sad.

CHAPTER EIGHT

TESTING TIMES

My Obsessive Compulsive Disorder and my other problems certainly would make for testing times ahead, and I also had another test of a different time ahead. For my university course, I had to do a dissertation. This was a totally new experience for me. I had never done one before and I knew that whilst I had plenty of time to get it right, if I got it wrong, I would throw away all of the other work I had done on the course, and the whole year would have been wasted. On the upside, as I began work on it I received the confirmation that I had passed all of the other modules I had undertaken on my course, so I knew that I didn't have any retakes to do. Also on the upside, I had found a good topic to do for my dissertation. I set about gathering information from various sources, including managing to get interviews from various libraries in order to find out how they had thought the internet had affected them. Things went well, but that was the upside.

On the downside, before I had started work on the dissertation I had left Loughborough for a couple of weeks to look after a house for some close friends for whilst they went on holiday. There was no problem with this, but when I got back to Loughborough I found that the first year students who had been living in the halls of residence directly next to my flat had gone home for the summer, and some oriental students staying in Loughborough over the summer had moved in there. I had no objection whatsoever to them being there, I was just scared out of my mind that I would meet them on the stairs of the halls of residence and accidentally blurt out something racist or inappropriate that they would take quite rightly offence at and complain. Another problem which my OCD had given me was that (as discussed in the previous chapter) when I was out in the town or on the campus, I would be scared that I would blurt out inappropriate language that busted its way into my head and said itself over and over again. When I would get back to the privacy of my flat I would try and work out if I said or just thought these evil words by saying them out loud and try and remember if I had heard myself say those words whilst I had been outside. I found this system, whilst far from perfect helped me relax and reassure me that I had not said any racist words. The problem now was that I thought the walls of my flat were quite thin, and now that I had new people living next door, what if they heard something I said and thought I was talking

THE MINDSET OF A MENTAL PATIENT

about them?

I know that to many people reading this that these problems and actions I took might seem weird and stupid, but in my state, to me they seemed very real and worrying and I had to do it in order to try and stop myself worrying about them all of the time, which was not easy. In honesty, this behaviour caused as many worries as it solved, and certainly didn't make things any happier or improve anything. It never did work, but every time I tried it, I stupidly thought it might. Three of the poems I wrote at this time show how confused and angry I was with myself for carrying out these stupid safety behaviours which in the long run were just keeping me paranoid and frightened that I would get into trouble and be thrown of the course because people thought that I was a racist:

Sanity departs
And paranoia cheers,
Now it's back in control
Inside my mind's fears.
Trying to shake it,
Yelling in fear.

Does nothing at all
Except engage the reverse gear,
Permanently going backwards
At a breakneck pace,
Revisiting the regrets
That litter my race.
Sighing, trying, and wishing I was dying.

115

Moping and panicking,
Years spent crying,

Making something out of nothing,
Interpreting events wrong.
Never stopping from my backwards journey,
Destroying myself with a con.

Finding no way out,
Onwards goes this black,
Revolving around my raging brain,
Ever refusing to change tack.
Valueless minds like mine go to hell,
Ever since confidence,
Reeled from our lives and fell.

Darker than this poem was another, which I wrote,
in a similar style to 'The Agony' from chapter five.
It is one of the darkest and most bitter poems I
have ever written. As had happened too many
times in my previous workplace, the rug was
always pulled from under my feet, just when things
appeared to be getting better. Every time, the
Devil was laughing at me from inside my head
when it all went wrong. He knew the pain he was
causing me. He would not leave me alone. I
believed it was him who was controlling all of the
negative emotions in me, such as the fear, the
paranoia and the depression. On one night when
the rug had been pulled from under me once
again, I wrote this in a fit of unbridled
hopelessness and depression:

THE MINDSET OF A MENTAL PATIENT

So This is It

Is this it?
The sum total of my life.
A dizzy haze of badly conceived ideas
To try and find out if I've offended?

Two diseases conspire to make me paranoid and
unacceptable,
Not least to myself.

An Obsessive Compulsive Disorder
Scares me that I am spouting racist insults,
Against others that live near.

What is this pain on my shoulder?
It is overbearing paranoia.
"You really said that," it says,
"You didn't just imagine it.
They will complain and you will be in trouble.
They will not believe you reasons.
You will be shamed out of existence when you
were so close your goal.

I have pulled the rug from under your feet,
Like I have done so often before,
And then I giggle at your misfortune
As again you fall flat on the floor.

I have done it so often,
I will do it again,
I think up new plans inside my den,

For it is so comfortable in your broken brain,
(For me not for you that is)
For you it's always the same.

I enjoy tinkering with your mind's controls
To do this and that,
All to the same conclusion,
That you'll fall right hard down BLAT!
And as you are floundering and you head feels so sore,
I send twisted thoughts and possibilities
To chill you to a worried core.

But enough of my vibrant rhythms,
So to bed I must rest,
But there will be no sleep for you, my friend,
As you worry about my next plan to put you to the test."

So this is it,
The sum total of my life.
Each day trying to live on my wits,
But scared witless about all the offence I might have caused,
Which haunts me in any second when my brain it is paused.

My brain is so hungry,
It eats up my soul,
And when that's gone,
Its hunger pangs are like rumbles of thunder,
Heralding the impending doom,
Blanking out the light into the gloom.

THE MINDSET OF A MENTAL PATIENT

But what will happen?
The fear is almost as bad as the fear happening,
Until the fear happens when it will seem 10 times
worse.
For the rest of my existence will I live with this
curse?
Will I live with it?
Will I die with it?
Will I scare off a potential bride with it?
No one will ever want me after this.
So its 60 years and counting,
With my paranoia sprouting,
Endless new ways in which to take the piss.

Yes, this is it,
The sum total of my life,
With Asperger's and OCD,
Who plunge knives into my brain
And twist them so thinking straight is impossible,
Creating a man who cannot interact with anyone,
Without being sacked from being a friend or being
a lover.
It will always be like this.
Why do I bother?

Yes, this is it.
My sum total's not alive.
Death, please knock me out,
The fight's yours,
I'll take a dive.

And finally, after another black occasion when I

was walking home after a bad day on the campus, I passed a Chinese man as I was about to get back to the relative safety of my flat, and an evil racist insult flashed at high volume though my brain, and I was almost certain that I had said it. In frustration, anger and desperation I wrote the following poem to the Devil. I *knew* now that it was he who was trying to make my life unlivable. This was quite close to the end of my course, and I was now frightened stiff that I would get into trouble for what I thought had happened (when in fact it hadn't), and that I might be thrown off the course so close to my goal. I could have given it all up, but I decided to stay and fight, just to let the Devil know that he was not going to get me that easily:

Inside the Mind of World War III

Hell is raging in my head,
With all hope's soldiers lying dead,
As again, my OCD commits its deadly deed,
And again my shattered happiness
Is machine-gunned down to bleed.

Will I recover this time only to be sent back to the front?
And just be battered down in battle by an instrument that is blunt.
Conscripted into mental illness,
Each day I'm forced to fight,
On life's frightening bloody battlefield,
Before I can briefly rest each night.

THE MINDSET OF A MENTAL PATIENT

And when each next day's battle commences on
life's battlefield,
Hell's angels are given the order to charge,
And I feel my fate is sealed,
As they surround my last few soldiers of hope,
And beat them up into a pulp,
I fear the day when they will all be gone,
And then all I will do is gulp,
For then the Devil will move in for the kill
On all people like me who are mentally ill.

Because for our brains there is no quick-fix
mender,
But I'll tell you now Satan:
"I will never surrender!"
Because I'd rather live and fight for what seems a
hopeless cause,
Than take the easy way out and become one of
yours,
Hell on earth is better than hell in hell.
The problems you've sent me I've seen all before,
And although they depress me and make me sad
to the core
And make me feel bad to the power of three,
I tell you now Satan:
"YOU DON'T GET ME!

Through all your planned fears,
You've been trying for years
To get me to jump into a fire and brimstone grave.
My life might be hell,
But my soul I won't sell,

I will never be your eternal slave."

For I know that life is just a test,
So I know that must try my best to weather the
dark storms
That create my hell on earth,
For if I can get through them now,
I know that I will win and how!
And look forward to Heaven and my real birth.

So on life's frightening bloody battlefield,
Where I've been injured and I've reeled,
Shot down in the tests of life,
But I'm not yet dead.

It's true that my life is no fun,
Being burnt by the dark side of the sun,
And the new dawn of every day I always dread.

But each day as my battered heartbeat soars,
I'll keep on fighting for my hopeless cause,
That being to be demobbed from my mental
conscription.
And have a life on Civvy Street that tastes
altogether a bit more sweet,
Before a life in Heaven with no happiness
restriction.

The last few pages have been incredibly dark in
tone, and apologies if you have found any of the
words contain here unnerving, so I will now
change direction.

THE MINDSET OF A MENTAL PATIENT

In order to lighten the mood at this point I would like to tell you a story, which led to me writing a much lighter poem. As my time in Loughborough came towards its end, I started applying for jobs, and I was offered an interview in Swindon at two days notice. I had never been to Swindon before and I decided to use public transport to get there. I telephoned National Rail Enquiries, who said the cheapest ticket they could give me costed £100, which was rather expensive, so I phoned a coach company, who said they could do it for £50. No contest!

The coach left Loughborough at 4 A.M., but due to a breakdown, it was half an hour late arriving. In addition to this there were road works on the M1 going into London, (where my connecting coach left from), and we ended up hitting Central London in the middle of the morning rush hour! However, the driver was still keen to make up time, and so dodged through the traffic at high speed, I felt rather scared, thinking we were going to crash! In the end I decided to keep my eyes shut, that way, I reasoned, that if there was a pile up, I couldn't be called as a witness! Fortunately, we arrived in London in one piece.

After the interview in Swindon and an equally hair-raising journey back to a London coach station later that evening, whilst I was waiting for my connecting coach back to Loughborough, I wrote this poem:

Christopher J. Fairweather

The Cavalier Coach Drivers of London Town

The Cavalier Coach drivers of old London Town,
When it comes to scaring passengers, they win
the crown.
Through the gaps in the traffic with precision they
slide,
Leaving just millimeters between the cars on
either side.

If I had an clout with the transport powers,
Their job would be the new white-knuckle ride out
at Alton Towers.

People could pay to be scared for their lives,
And be taken on one of these breakneck speed
drives,
Through the capital and all its tight passes,
Hoping the drivers' remembered his glasses.

In terror for cover under their seats they'd dive,
Hoping they'll come out of the experience alive.
But it would be much cheaper I must confess,
If you booked a coach to London, it would cost
you much less!

Then all the terror you can experience for real.
Try not to have a coronary,
Yes, that's the deal!
As they dodge past the taxis in their dark shades
of black,
Through the streets of London,
With gay abandon they attack,

THE MINDSET OF A MENTAL PATIENT

All other motorists and pedestrians too,
And for the ultimate thrill-seekers,
Here's the challenge for you!

Take to the streets of London by bike,
That experience will scare you as much as you
like.
For when the speeding coach driver bears down
on your tail,
You'll wish you were traveling in London by rail!

So no more roller coasters for you with no fears,
Go by coach for the most frightening time of your
living years!

My final two weeks in Loughborough passed
reasonably uneventfully, the worries were still
there, but not as bad as they had been. Finally,
the hand in date for my dissertation arrived. I took
it in and thanked my supervisor for all her help,
and I would like to take this opportunity to thank
the people who helped me whilst I was at
Loughborough University, staff and friends. In
particular, my supervisor for being so helpful to me
with my dissertation, to the lady responsible for
offering me a place on the course to begin with, to
all the lectueres and of coruse the medical staff for
keeping me mentally in a much better frame of
mind than I would have been without them, and of
course to my small circle of friends, and everyone
else who helped me along the way. I am sorry if
sometimes I seemed rather strange, but if you are
reading this book, hopefully you will understand

more as to why I was the way I was.

Now all I had to do was wait for my results. The nervous weeks passed, and eventually the date came around. I checked my university email. I HAD PASSED! I had come to the campus mentally ill, been diagnosed with Asperger's Syndrome and taken on an Obsessive Compulsive Disorder, BUT I HAD COME OUT ON TOP!

....

That is the end of my story, and I would like to thank you for taking the time to read it. I admit it has been rather dark, and I know I have come across as a rather strange person, but the point I am trying to make is that, in spite of all my problems, I have led a close to normal life. I am not trying to boast when I say what I am about to say, but it is true. Since going to university for the first time in 1998, I have gained a BA (Hons) degree in Business Administration, which took three years of my life. During this time, I held part-time employment. After I had finished my course, I held a full time job for two and a half years before returning to university and gaining an MA in Information and Library Management, and during all of this time, I have suffered from mental health problems of one sort or another. On the way through, I have met prejudiced people and employers, and by contrast, people who were happy to help me and be friends despite my problems. I would like to say a big thank you to all of you who have helped me. What I am trying to say is, if I (a man of average intelligence) am capable of the above, there are many other people with mental health problems who are capable of doing the same, and this brings me on to the final point of this book. All that now remains is for me to find a job, and this is where the trouble can lie.

Some weeks after I had left Loughborough I was watching BBC News 24 on National Mental Health Day, which they had various items about. They reeled of various rather disturbing statistics and stories about how people with mental health problems are often (though it must be said not always) treated by employers and prospective employers. I wrote a poem about these statistics:

Facts and Figures

Some facts and figures about us
With problems with mental health,

2/3 of employers will not employ us,
Just by using stealth.

It's catch-22 when we fill in the application form.
If we declare mental health problems
It won't go down a storm,
But if we don't and then they do find out,
They will sack us for not telling,
And won't care about the doctor's reports,
Sent to their office dwelling.

Christopher J. Fairweather

And yet 1 in 4 of us will have mental health
problems
At some point in our lives,
But mental health problems are one of the things
Employers can still stigmatise
Without any form of remorse at all,
Still with a conscience with no dent,
Even though the figure of those who suffer is 25%.

Just because they can't see it,
They think they have the right,
To hound us with the problems,
Right into the night,
And thinking we're all psychos in all but name,
They wipe us out of their employment frame.

So we have to put up with their prejudiced side,
For the spectrum of mental health problems
Is broad and it is wide,
And in spite of our problems
Most of us work very well,
But obviously 2/3 of employers have only heard
tell
Of those with the worst problems,
(For I admit they are there),
As they look at our application forms
With their prejudiced stare,
For we had these conditions
In DNA from birth.

But 2/3 of employers
Refuse to let us prove out worth.

CHAPTER NINE

A FEW LIGHTER (AND A FEW NOT SO LIGHT) ASIDES

Through some of my period of writing poems I have written some totally unconnected with my mental state. Some are intended to be funny, and whilst a few of them are in the main chapters of this book, here are some which whilst I did not think comfortably fitted into the main book itself, I still thought deserved to be included.

This first one concerns the topic of newsreaders, one of them in particular. Moira Stewart reading the news is one of my first memories of television, (circa 1981) and in around 2004 I noticed the following situation:

The Beauty Secrets of Moira Stewart

I wish I knew the beauty secrets of Moira Stewart. I keep wondering, "How does that woman do it?" She's read the news on television since I was three,

And hasn't aged one iota over time as I can see.

She could make a fortune, not reading the news,
But endorsing beauty products for others to choose.
Her methods must be more effective than what's tested on mice,
With her you'd become twice as attractive, and for half the price.
Because what she uses must be better than L'Oreal or Maybeline.
She could make a fortune out there on the fashion scene.

But instead, she did the decent thing and she read the news,
Which was a far more worthwhile job than advertising vile face cream goos.
She hasn't sold out for an easy buck,
Or been a surgeon's model for the latest nip and tuck.
She done something useful with her life throughout her living years,
So for her integrity we should all give three cheers.

So, for the beauty conscious there who want to know how to do it,
Don't spend a fortune on cosmetic s, just ask Moira Stewart!

Next, a little poem about Murphy's Law. This is a subject my father taught me about when I was young, many years later; I wrote this poem about it.

Murphy's Law

This man Murphy must love his work,
As from his obligations he'll never shirk,
As he finds it fun
In the short and long run,
To work all the time,
Instead of lying in the sun.

But if he did lie out there
We'd be all the more happy,
As we wouldn't be bothered by this little chappy,
Who enjoys engineering things so life won't run smooth,
Though he and his company are forever in the groove.

He must have a company for one simple reason,
As doing what he does for the world every season,
Must take more than one man to get it all done,
And so with chosen others, he will share his fun.

Which idiotic Government passed Murphy's Law?
They had an odd sense of humor,
Of that, I'm sure.
For whilst most of the time it's not too annoying,
Without Murphy, we could live life.
With a bit more enjoying.

This limerick was written after I saw one Boris

Johnson's hilarious attempts at presenting Have I Got News for You.

Boris Johnson

The bumbling buffoon Boris Johnson,
Was brought up by ants in Wisconsin.
He helped build their nest
With a decaying string vest,
But was then squashed by old Charles Bronson.

We have all heard the urban myth orange is the only word in the English language that does not rhyme with anything. After I heard this pseudo-statistic, for reasons I cannot fathom I suddenly started to wonder that, if orange is the only word that rhymes with nothing else, every other word must rhyme with something else, and what would rhyme with Natterjack?... Crackerjack was the only word I could think of!

These two words stayed in my brain, and one day on a lunch break at work, I finally found the inspiration to write this meaningless piece of nonsense (which probably won't mean anything to anyone born after 1985, in which case please fell free to rejoin the rest of us at last paragraph of the next page. For older readers, feel free to join them, and either way, turn the page now...

THE MINDSET OF A MENTAL PATIENT

Natterjack Crackerjack

A toad who was Natterjack
Appeared on Crackerjack,
Like all Natterjack toads do.
Said the producer of Crackerjack
To the toad who was Natterjack,
"Are you wild or do you live in a zoo?"
Said the toad who was Natterjack
To the producer of Crackerjack,
"What business is that of yours?"
Said the producer of Crackerjack
To the toad (Natterjack),
"I'm researching the species of yours,
To see if toads that are Natterjack
There is one great big lack
Due to killing against nature's laws.
That is why I of Crackerjack
Investigate Natterjack."
Said the toad,
"Good luck with your cause!"

So the toad who was Natterjack
Appeared on Crackerjack,
And won fair and square
And by right,
And the producer of Crackerjack found
Of toads, there's no lack
And the future of the species looks bright.

This is another piece of nonsense about a story I
heard (I know not if it was true) that Ken
Livingstone was banning bendy buses on the

grounds that they could spontaneously combust.

Bendy Buses

A spontaneously combustible bendy bus
Is made of the material for an elephant's truss.
So when Red Ken has taken them away,

We should know what to use them for,
I say.

We could help old elephants
Live that much longer,
And then they could make their communities
stronger,
By passing on more knowledge
From the old to the young,
And teaching the evils of staying out in the sun.
For as elephants get older
They get wiser you see.
They could invent sun block Factor 203,
Which could help human beings
Who get lost in the Sahara,
For as long as they had water
They could walk that much farther,
Without getting sun burnt,
It's clever you see.
That's what elephants could do for you and me.

So there's a future in Bendy Buses,
Don't throw them away.
They'll help elephants save lives,
So let them show the way.

THE MINDSET OF A MENTAL PATIENT

Since I was young, I have loved the animations of Oliver Postgate, particularly Bagpuss, and The Clangers. I am frequently critical of some television today, and the quality of some of today's children's programmes, combined with the high-pressure advertising and merchandising that goes with them led me to write this next piece.

Postgate's Mice

Do children learn from modern cartoons?
No.
What do they learn from modern Newsround?
Woe.
Given the choice, I'd go backing a trice,
To Oliver Postgate and his moon-based mice.

Trumpton, Chigley and Camberwick Green.
There was something to learn
In those programmes we'd seen.
Songs to remember,
Morals, etc.
How to care for animals,
Like Blue Peter's Petra.

But now we're stuck
With the Teletubbies, sadly,
Who simply teach English to children, badly.
Given the choice I'd go back in a trice,
To Bagpuss and Yaffle,
And the organ-based mice.

But now we have high-pressure advertising
And masses of Christmas merchandising,
And all of a sudden, the programme comes
second
As the profits of the toys and the posters are
reckoned.
Entertaining and teaching the kids 'aint enough,
We have to force-feed them this second-rate stuff,
And make them think
That in order to look really cool
They need mountains of this stuff
To take daily to school.

Where will all this merchandising lead?
Shouldn't we be teaching the evils of greed?
Given the choice, I'd go back in a trice,
To the sense and simplicity of all Postgate's mice.

Since I first saw her on the late-night current
affairs programme, The Sundays, in 1998, I have
been a huge fan of the late, great and much
missed comedian Linda Smith. I saw her perform
at the Nuffield Theatre in Southampton once, and
she was hilarious. I met her afterwards and she
was just as warm and friendly off-stage as she
was on.

I remember I came back to my flat in
Loughborough one evening and switched on BBC
News 24 just in time to hear the news that she had
died of cancer. She had told very few people that
she was ill, and it was a shock to the nation. That
night I wrote this little poem as a way of thanking

THE MINDSET OF A MENTAL PATIENT

her for all the pleasure she had brought me, and countless others.

So-long Linda

So-long Linda,
Now you've gone,
And although the world still carries on,
It won't be the same
Now you can't do the biz,
On Just a Minute,
Or The News Quiz.

'Britain's wittiest person
Of 2002,'
We'll keep that title safe for you,
For it's sad that you cannot win it again.
You were a better entertainer
Than most other men.

Time wasting was simply a pleasure with you,
As was I'm Sorry I Haven't a Clue,
And I'd like to say thank you for 2003,
When you signed my Just a Minute tape cover for me.

So, so-long Linda,
Now you're not here
To entertain us with your brand of cheer,
But we'll keep thinking of you
For a long time to come,
Now that your life,
On this planet is done.

This next poem is one of my favorites. Again, it is a piece of nonsense, and let it be a cautionary tale to anyone thinking of going out to rob a bank.

A Cautionary Tale

Please listen while I tell you the cautionary tale
Of Julian Guillemot-Slate.
He did his best to hold up the Old Glasgow Bank,
But sadly collapsed under the weight.

The Old Bill was called
And a crowd was enthralled,
(Well, half interested at any rate),
As they jacked up the bank
From whence it had sank,
And pulled Guillemot out
In his squashed flattened state.

He was hauled up in Court
In the seaside resort of Brise-Norton,
(The birthplace of toast),
And the judge sent him down
With a world-weary frown,
To the prison which they'd built on the coast.

But Guillemot-Slate
Though as flat as a plate,
Would not wait for his sentence to pass.
He planned to escape
With a plan second rate.
(The underhanded snake-in-the-grass).

THE MINDSET OF A MENTAL PATIENT

He slipped through his cell bars
On to two passing cars,
Being towed by a transporter truck.
"I'm free now," he thought,
As he left the resort...
… But I'm afraid he was right out of luck.

For the cars were being towed
To the dump up the road,
Which had a crusher for crushing old metal,
Such as cars and the like,
And the odd motorbike,
To make new things all fine and fettle.

And Guillemot-Slate had left it too late
As he was squashed out of all shape and form,
Now combined with the metal,
(The wrong place to settle),
And now poetic justice
Was just about to storm.

For the metal was taken to Lord Kevin Dacon
At the National Pound Coin Minting Factory.
"Prepare the coin mould," the Foreman was told,
"For this metal is just satisfactory",
"We'll melt it down first so the impurities burst
And then lots of pound coins we will make.
I know where to send them,
It's a nice place that lends them,
It's the Old Glasgow Bank by the lake!"

Guillemot-Slate was appalled at his fate,

That was the one place that he'd tried to rob.
And now it will be his home until he's called for a loan,
From mow on that will be his job.
And so ends my tale of Guillemot-Slate,
To find if he'd be lent out,
He'd just have to wait.
But no matter how things turn out now,
It's all his own fault,
As he resides now as coins,
In the Glasgow Bank's vault.

This final poem I wrote about my dear grandmother who I was very close to. She lived in Norfolk, and the many times I went to see her on holidays were some of the happiest of my life. She died unexpectedly in 2000, and I miss her to this day. This poem is about the happy times I had with her, and how I believe it is true that the simple pleasures are the best.

The Last Game of Scrabble

The last game of Scrabble,
The last round of Golf,
And the last time we watched
Animal Hospital with Rolf.

The last time I saw you,
Everything was fine,
And I wish I could see you again right now,
As the funeral bells they chime.

THE MINDSET OF A MENTAL PATIENT

The last thing that you did for me
Was the most important yet.
But it won't be the last thing,
You ever do for me I bet.
I know you're watching over me,
In your place of eternal rest.
I hope to see you there one day,
And I will if I try my best.
But I need your help to lead my life,
To get to you at the end,
Which will be the beginning of eternity,
For you and I my friend.

The last game is never there,
We can play forever more,
If I can just get through my life,
And open Heaven's door.

The next game of Scrabble,
And the next round of golf,
And the next time we watch
Animal Hospital with Rolf,
Will be the sweetest things that happen
When I'm on the other side,
When once again together,
On cloud nine we can ride.

Post Script

Recently, I listened to a programme on Radio 4, which highlighted to me a reason why my brain works in such an idiosyncratic fashion. Inside my brain there is too much of a certain chemical. It is called:

Dopamine

I've found out today that Dopamine,
Is why I am who I am.
Its formulated in my being
Since my first day in my pram.

Over-production of Dopamine,
Inside my middle-brain,
Can make me seem so strange to others,
Who wonder if I'm sane.

I don't give three cheers for Dopamine,
For it has no regret.
It has drowned out reason in my mind,
I haven't found the exit yet.

Dopamine is the chemical blindfold,
So I cannot see sense,
But I can feel the paranoia it brings,
And remain permanently tense.

THE MINDSET OF A MENTAL PATIENT

Dopamine
Operates
Permanently
Everyday
Riling
Me
Inside
Nastily.
Every night
It leaves me in fright.
It's merciless,
It's dastardly.

But I am thankful I have to say,
To know the chemical reason
Why I'm this way,
Before, when I didn't (And that time was long),
I did not know why I felt so wrong.

So whilst my problems are not solved,
I say it's nice to know finally the reason why
I have felt so low.

It's true in Dopamine my brain does drown,
Holding my face in a permanent frown.

But thankfully as I found out today,
From Radio 4 via electric cable,
How I might be able to develop new skills,
So on Dopamine I can turn the table.

Thank you to all who know me.
This where the story really starts…

Lightning Source UK Ltd.
Milton Keynes UK
26 October 2009

145410UK00001BA/6/P